AGING
Reframed

A WORKBOOK FOR FINDING YOUR PEACE, ENERGY, AND POWER IN MID-LIFE

SUSAN REYNOLDS

chartwell
books

Quarto

This edition published in 2025 by Chartwell Books,
an imprint of The Quarto Group
142 West 36th Street, 4th Floor
New York, NY 10018 USA
T (212) 779-4972
www.Quarto.com

10 9 8 7 6 5 4 3 2 1

Chartwell titles are also available at discount for retail, wholesale, promotional, and bulk purchase. For details, contact the Special Sales Manager by email at specialsales@quarto.com or by mail at The Quarto Group, Attn: Special Sales Manager, 100 Cummings Center Suite 265D, Beverly, MA 01915, USA.

ISBN: 978-0-7858- 4691-8

Publisher: Wendy Friedman
Publishing Director: Meredith Mennitt
Editor: Joanne O'Sullivan
Designer: Brianna Tong
Image credits: Shutterstock

Printed in Malaysia

This book provides general information. It should not be relied upon as recommending or promoting any specific diagnosis or method of treatment for a particular condition. It is not intended as a substitute for medical advice or for direct diagnosis and treatment of a medical or psychological condition by a qualified physician or therapist. Readers who have questions about a particular condition, possible treatments for that condition, or possible reactions from the condition or its treatment should consult a career counselor, or physician, therapist, or other qualified healthcare professional.

CONTENTS

Aging with Intention

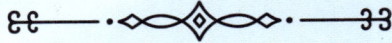

&& — ·◇◇◇◇◇· — 33

Hopefully you experienced a healthy, supportive childhood and a stimulating and success-filled young adulthood. If so, you're likely riding high in your middle years, feeling alert, strong, healthy, vibrant, and enthusiastic about life, as well you should be. However, there will come a time—not so long from now—when you notice that your body and your brain have begun to change. Some of the changes will be improvements: You'll be more knowledgeable, more confident, more thoughtful and measured, and often more empathetic and generous. Though they will come slowly, almost imperceptibly at first, some of the changes will not be so welcome. Over time, you'll lose strength, energy, velocity, and even brainpower. We're not telling you this to frighten you, but there is no denying that you will grow old, *if you're lucky!*

The truth is that you have the power to make changes *now* that will maximize the positive aspects of future changes, minimize any detrimental changes, and help you become healthier and happier as you age. Facing the future with courage and making changes that will benefit your aging process now and as you age gracefully will contribute greatly to keeping you healthy, active, strong, alert, vibrant, and enthusiastic well into your nineties.

You can indeed age gracefully, particularly if you focus on creating and sustaining an *active, intentional journey* focused on three primary needs:

- To maintain your overall health and physical function
- To maintain your cognitive functions (processing, memory, decision-making, etc.)
- To stay involved in social activities and productive pursuits.

While worrying about getting old is neither wise, nor useful, preparing yourself to age gracefully is essential to maximizing and enjoying your golden years. Studies have shown that those who have, or develop, the healthiest habits in their forties, fifties, and sixties are the ones who are far more likely to remain healthy and active into their seventies, eighties, and nineties.

In this book, we're going to cover the strategies you need to create the kinds of healthy habits that will help you age gracefully, all while enjoying peace, energy, and power now, and well into your future. We'll begin by noting that the best strategy is a holistic approach, integrating mindset, physical health, cognitive vitality, social connections, and planning. And the best way to gear yourself up for being a healthy, strong, vibrant, high-functioning octogenarian is to get started *now*.

All you have to do is to turn the page and jump in.

"I'm super-conscious that I'm closer to death. But it doesn't really bother me that much—what bothers me is that my body is basically not mine! My knees are not mine, my hips are not mine, my shoulder's not mine. You're looking at somebody who's only me from here (my neck) up…The fact that I'm still alive and working, wow! Who cares if I still don't have my old joints and can't ski or bike or run anymore? You can be old at sixty, and really young at eighty-five."

— JANE FONDA

GET A
New
Attitude

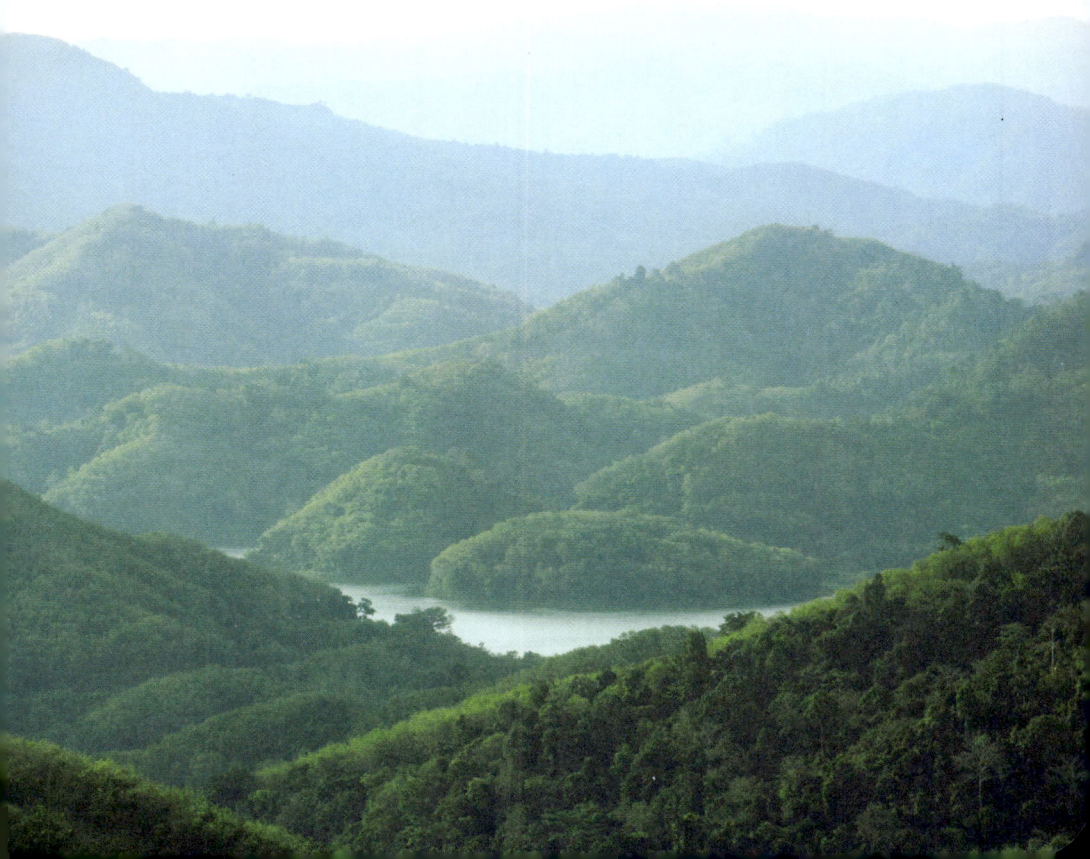

Get a New Attitude

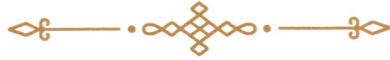

Across a variety of measures (including incidence of diseases, mortality rates, cognitive function, physical strength), people today are not aging *more* but are simply aging *more slowly*. According to statistics compiled by the American Psychological Association, one out of every four sixty-five-year-olds today will live past age ninety, and one out of ten will live past age ninety-five. The number of Americans over age eighty-five is increasing faster than for any other age group. Today's *average* life expectancy is 84.3 years for men and 86.6 years for women.

The fact that we are living longer compels us to reframe how we live. Given that you'll likely have a lot more time, you should avoid basing your perspective on your own future on what you have heard about or observed in the past. Reframing how you think about aging will help you live a longer, healthier, happier, and more productive life.

Aging Reframed will help you take a fresh look at your current mental, physical, and social well-being, offering you a chance to reflect and reset. You'll learn how to reframe your thinking to embrace the aging process, adjust your habits to reinforce health, nourish and protect your body and brain, and find the purpose and meaning that will make your latter years some of the best of your life. You'll discover how you can create and bolster social networks, and plan ahead for a long, happy, healthy, productive, and fulfilling life—right up to the end.

Let's get started by talking about common misconceptions about aging.

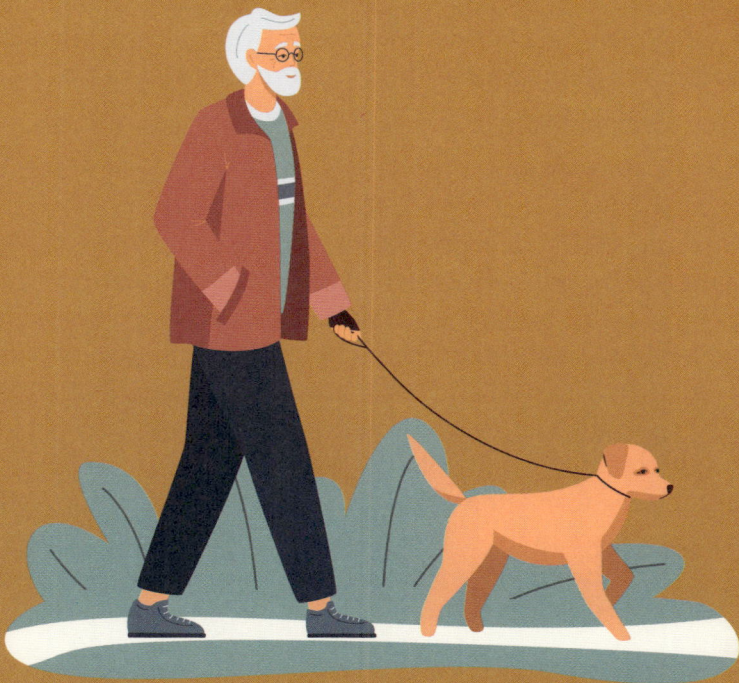

"AARP reminds us that aging is something to embrace, a badge of honor, actually. As the author of *The Little Prince* put it, 'In spite of decoys, jolts, and ruts, you have continued to plod like a horse, drawing a cart.' And I'm so fortunate I am still here, still drawing my cart. Well, I may be entering the winter of my career, but the view is anything but bleak; against the glittering snow, vibrant, pink, red plum blossoms bloom—a flower you can't find in any other season."

— JOAN CHEN

COMMON MISCONCEPTIONS ABOUT AGING

No matter how old you are, you have likely experienced age bias. When you're younger, you're presumed to be naïve, immature, unreliable. In middle age, you might be considered career-driven, selfish, myopic, overburdened. When you're older, you are often viewed as frail, forgetful, uninteresting, set in your ways, or dependent.

According to the United States Census Bureau, the number of Americans aged sixty-five and older is projected to double from 46 million to more than 98 million by 2060. It will be the first time in history that the number of older adults outnumbers children under age five. This demographic shift has moved the focus of researchers, health care providers, and policymakers from how to extend the lifespan to how to improve the quality of our later years. Staying healthy, active, and productive are admirable goals for our nation's older adults. However, society's view of 'old age' has not always kept up with the reality of being old in America. Many current beliefs about aging are based on information garnered by looking too far into the past or observing older generations. That's no longer valid. Today, there's much more focus on healthy eating habits, exercise, and self-care, and advances in medical research and health care have conquered maladies that used to shorten life.

"My movie career didn't begin in earnest until I was fifty years old. These last thirty years have been the best of my life, and I've learned a lot on this journey."

— MORGAN FREEMAN

The attitudes that underlie age bias are often rooted in falsehoods. Becca Levy, PhD and professor of epidemiology and psychology at Yale School of Public Health, uses fact-checking to chip away at age stereotypes. In her recent book, *Breaking the Age Code: How Your Beliefs About Aging Determine How Long and Well You Live*, she took aim at more than a dozen beliefs about getting older. "In every case, I found information that not only contradicted the negative stereotype but also highlighted a strength that comes with aging," she said, as reported in an article she authored about ageism on the American Psychological Association website (3/23). Some of these beliefs include the following.

Older people experience a steep decline in health. While it is true that the risk of some chronic diseases and dementia increases with age, most older adults maintain quite good health and cognitive functioning.

People become less creative as they get older. Levy found a host of examples of artists and musicians who became more creative and more generative later in life.

All types of cognitive abilities inevitably worsen with age. It's true that some cognitive skills, such as reaction times, tend to slow a bit over time. But other functions remain robust and even improve. One study of older adults, for instance, showed they were better than middle-age adults at orienting their attention and ignoring distractions (*Veríssimo, J., et al., Nature Human Behaviour, Vol. 6, No. 1, 2022*).

As they age, many people suffer from depression. While depression often accompanies poor health, isolation, loneliness, and loss, many make healthy choices and create lifestyles that improve their health, bolster their connectivity, and stave off depression. In fact, according to what is called 'the aging paradox,' many people past age sixty-five are relatively happy, happier than they were in middle age, and often even happier than they were in their youth.

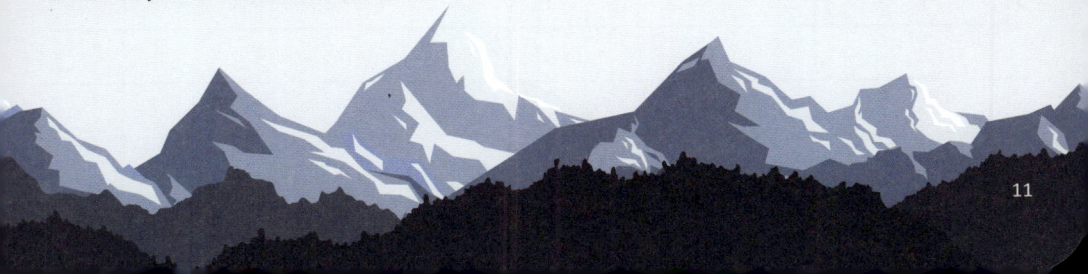

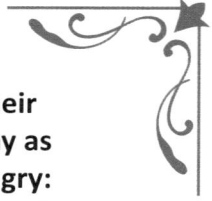

What negative biases might you hold regarding people in their seventies, eighties, and nineties? List at least ten, or as many as you can think of, and don't worry if they're dark or seem angry: you'll be reframing your attitude as you work through this book.

1 _____

_____

_____

2 _____

_____

_____

3 _____

_____

_____

4 _____

_____

_____

5 _____

_____

_____

6

_____

_____

_____

_____

7

_____

_____

_____

_____

8

_____

_____

_____

_____

9

_____

_____

_____

_____

10

_____

_____

_____

_____

Are any of the negative ideas you recorded true for all elderly people, or only true for a few people you might know? Why do you think you've made these negative assumptions?

_____

_____

_____

_____

_____

_____

_____

_____

_____

"The older you are, the more interesting you are as a character. There's a whole life history and knowledge of the world and self-possession that come from someone who has seen more. That experienced point of view is always more exciting. Yes, things may start to sag and shift, but the older you are, the wiser, the funnier, the smarter you are. You become more you."

— MELISSA MCCARTHY

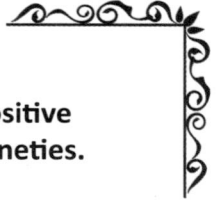

Based on facts you've learned thus far, write at least five positive statements about people in their seventies, eighties, and nineties.

1
_____

_____

_____

2
_____

_____

_____

3
_____

_____

_____

4
_____

_____

_____

5
_____

_____

_____

THE BENEFITS OF AGING

Although most middle-aged people bemoan the fact they're growing older, many of the benefits of aging are obvious. Think how far you've come since entering the world. You learned to walk, to talk, to read, to study, to make friends, to celebrate life, to take on responsibilities, to fall in love, perhaps to marry and have children, to nurture yourself and others, to advance in the larger world, and experience many wondrous things. You not only learned how to navigate the larger world, you likely settled upon and pursued a career, discovering plenty of friends along the way. These are all marvelous accomplishments, all of which have brought you to where you are now—older, wiser, and still full of fire. This doesn't have to change as you approach sixty, seventy, eighty, or ninety. Let's discuss the very real benefits of getting older.

As we age, we not only tend to become more agreeable and more conscientious but also tend to be better at regulating emotions. These positive changes often improve relationships, help us pay better attention to our health, and prevent us from entering risky situations.

Such changes may be partly responsible for another observed phenomenon, known as 'the paradox of aging.' As reported in an article on ageism on the American Psychological Association website (3/23), according to Karl Pillemer, PhD, a sociologist and professor of psychology and gerontology at Cornell University, "Older people tend to report greater happiness and life satisfaction compared to younger people."

Some researchers have debated the evidence for this so-called happiness curve, a U-shaped trend in which happiness levels are lowest in midlife. But in taking a comprehensive look at data from 145 countries, economist David Blanchflower concluded that, in fact, happiness sinks to a low-water mark in middle age before increasing again through later adulthood (*Journal of Population Economics*, Vol. 34, No. 2, 2021). Other research suggests that, contrary to popular belief, mental health also improves across the life span (Thomas, M. L., et al., *Journal of Clinical Psychiatry*, Vol. 77, No. 8, 2016). "This view that old age is all negative decline just doesn't seem to be the case," Pillemer said.

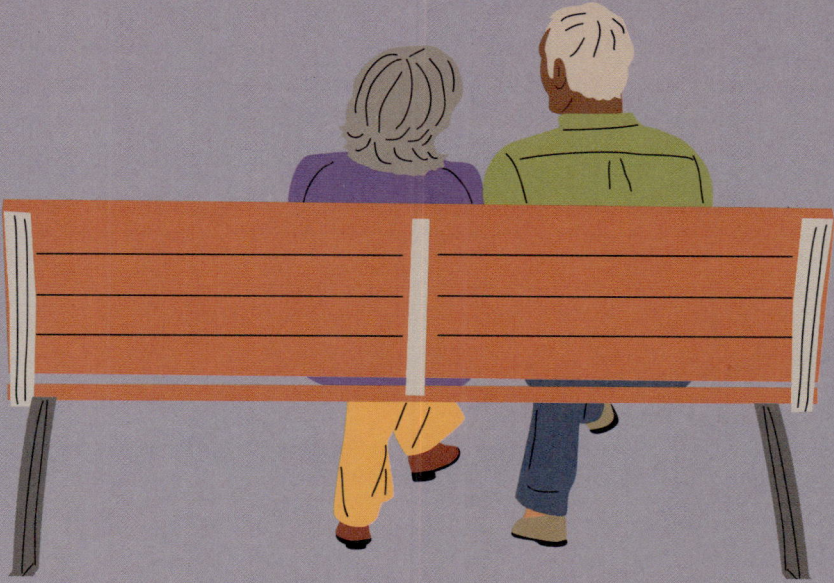

"Aging is not for the weak. One day you wake up and realize your youth is gone, but along with it, so go insecurity, haste, and the need to please . . . You learn to walk more slowly, but with greater certainty. You say goodbye without fear, and you cherish those who stay. Aging means letting go, it means accepting, it means discovering that beauty was never in our skin . . . but in the story we carry inside us."

— MERYL STREEP

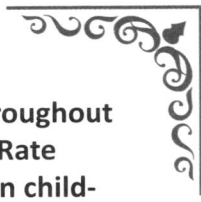

How do you feel about your levels of happiness throughout your life thus far? In childhood and as a teenager? Rate your levels of happiness in various stages, such as in childhood, in early adulthood, and in middle age, on a scale of 1-5, with five being 'very happy in general.'

Childhood (0-12)

1	2	3	4	5

Unhappy   Very Happy

Teenage Years (13-19)

1	2	3	4	5

Unhappy   Very Happy

Early Adulthood (20-40)

1	2	3	4	5

Unhappy   Very Happy

Middle Age (40-55)

1	2	3	4	5

Unhappy   Very Happy

Currently

1	2	3	4	5

Unhappy   Very Happy

What had the most effect on your level of happiness in each period?

_____

_____

_____

_____

During your happiest years, what did you do that specifically contributed to making them happy?

_____

_____

_____

_____

Are there steps you could take now to improve your level of happiness? What would those be?

_____

_____

_____

_____

What do you think will be most important to your personal happiness as you age? What can you do now to make those conditions likely to occur?

_____

_____

_____

_____

Misconceptions about how we age cognitively and how we feel about aging are rampant. Here are some basic facts.

- For most older adults, age-associated changes in cognition (thinking) are mild and do not significantly interfere with daily functioning.
- Older adults are capable of learning new skills even late in life, though learning may take longer than for younger adults.
- Short-term memory shows noticeable changes with age, but long-term memory declines less with age.
- Some changes in cognition are normal with age, such as slower reaction times and reduced problem-solving abilities. The speed with which information is encoded, stored, and retrieved also slows as we age. However, many older adults outperform their younger counterparts on intelligence tests that draw on accumulated knowledge and experience.
- Wisdom and creativity often continue to the very end of life. Some become even more creative.
- Personality traits remain relatively stable over time. For example, people who were outgoing during young adulthood are likely to be outgoing in later life.
- Most older adults report good mental health and have fewer mental health problems than other age groups.
- Dementia (including Alzheimer's disease, the most common type of dementia) is not a normal part of aging. Approximately 5 percent of individuals between seventy-one and seventy-nine and 37 percent of the population above ninety are affected.
- As they age, people are generally more satisfied with their lives and more optimistic about growing older.

This knowledge of current aging trends should help you reframe your thinking and develop a more positive view of aging.

"One of the strange things about adulthood is that you are your current self, but you are also all the selves you used to be, the ones you grew out of but can't ever quite get rid of."

— JOHN GREEN, *THE ANTHROPOCENE REVIEWED: ESSAYS ON A HUMAN-CENTERED PLANET*

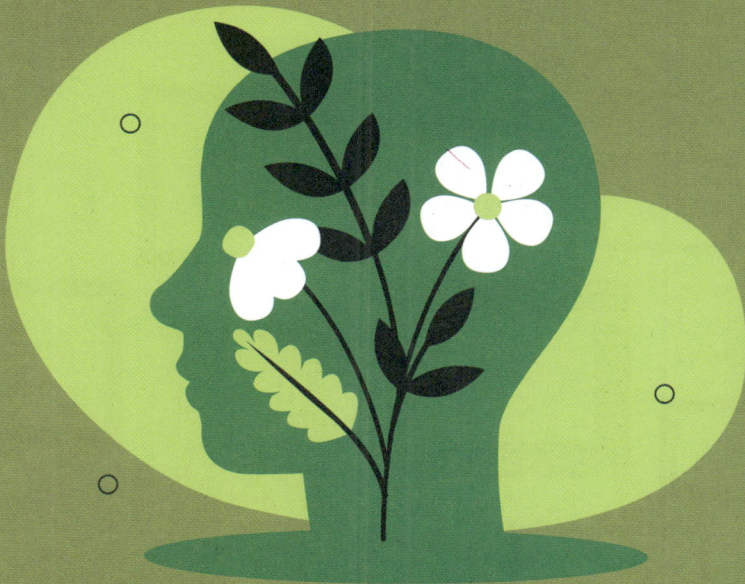

HOW TO COGNITIVELY REFRAME

We typically rely on our existing thoughts and beliefs when making choices. We frame according to our experiences and conclusions we've previously drawn. When *reframing*, we expand the parameters and consciously re-evaluate what we think or believe to see things in a new light. The value choices we make when reframing matter, as they not only affect how we move through life, but also how people will hear us, what they will understand, and how they will act towards us.

Cognitive reframing is a method that can help you identify, evaluate, and change unhelpful thought patterns. It can be an effective tool for addressing and overcoming cognitive distortions, or irrational thoughts that shape how you see yourself, others, and the world. Cognitive Behavioral Therapy (CBT), a therapeutic method commonly used to combat negative thinking, is one way you can shift your mindset and thereby learn to reframe, or learn to view a person, place, or situation from a different perspective. It's based on the idea that your *interpretation* of an event, rather than the actual event, determines your emotional reaction. Learning to reframe your perspective can lead to healthier outcomes. The process includes the following steps.

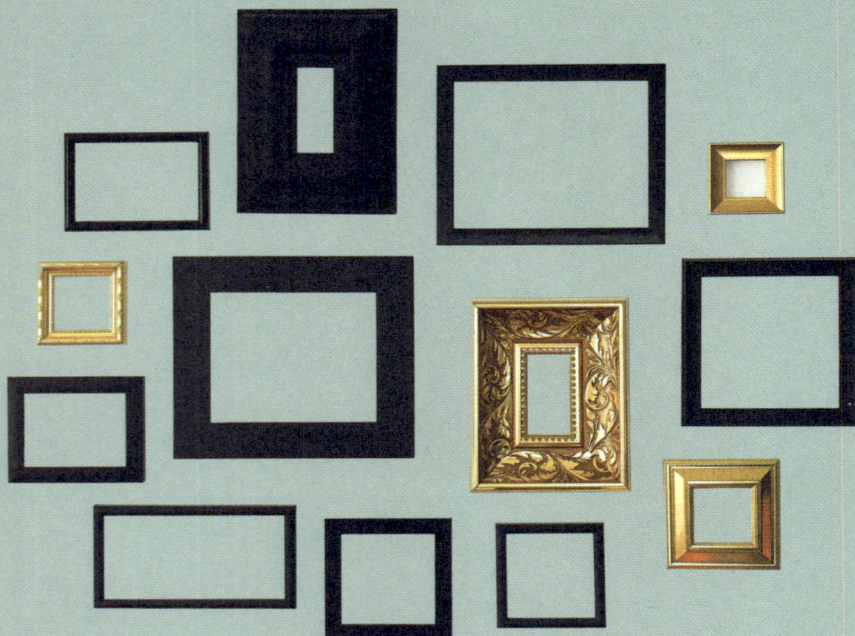

1. **Identify your thoughts.** Recognize unhelpful thought patterns and beliefs. These thoughts often involve cognitive distortions, such as overgeneralization, labeling, catastrophizing (always fearing the worst), and black-and-white thinking.

2. **Dispute your thoughts.** Once you identify an unhelpful thought, pause to ask yourself if there's any evidence to support it. Some questions to consider include:

    *   Am I being overreactive and/or jumping to conclusions?
    *   Am I biased? Are there other ways I could view the situation?
    *   Am I making it black or white instead of seeing complexity?
    *   Am I making faulty assumptions or seeing incorrectly?
    *   Could I be exaggerating or catastrophizing?
    *   What validates or refutes my response?
    *   Did I learn this from a reliable source?
    *   How would someone more objective think about the situation?
    *   Is my concern based more on how I *feel* than the facts of the situation?

3. **Replace your thoughts.** The goal is to replace unbalanced or unhelpful thoughts with more balanced and empowering alternatives. Use an example more relevant to your current life. Instead of thinking: "If I fail this job interview, I'll never succeed in my career." Obviously, going into any job interview would cause you to feel nervous and insecure, but if you paused to refute those ideas, you'd likely recognize that you are allowing your mind to generalize and your emotions to over-react. Once you refuted those thoughts, you could replace them with: "I'll prepare for the job interview so that I can feel confident that I'm presenting the best version of me."

In other words, you notice and refute negative thoughts that do not serve you and reframe the experience so you can see it in a positive light. The more you practice this, the more it will become second nature. Let's give it a try.

TRY REFRAMING

Think about a particularly strong negative thought you regularly have about aging that brings you down. What are the specifics within the thought (assumptions) that spark worry or fear about your own future? Really dig deep and dredge up linked thoughts that have created this view.

_____

_____

_____

_____

_____

_____

_____

_____

_____

_____

_____

_____

_____

_____

_____

_____

_____

_____

_____

_____

_____

_____

Now use the method you just learned to dispute your thought. Reviewing your own negative assumptions about aging, which ring true, and why?

_____

_____

_____

_____

Can you identify where you're getting caught up? Are you caught in black or white thinking? Are you biased? Exaggerating? Using faulty thinking? Refer to the list under "Dispute Your Thoughts" on page 23 to pinpoint where your cognitive processing is leading to negativity.

_____

_____

_____

_____

SHIFTING PERCEPTIONS

The 2024 German Aging Survey (involving 14,000 participants) found that people in their mid-sixties now define old age as starting around seventy-five, whereas a few decades ago, people of that age defined old age as starting around seventy-one (and sixty-five prior to that!). Researchers found that every increase in age you experience results in you moving the marker.

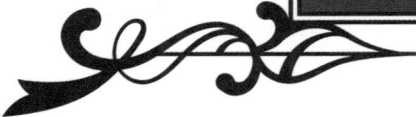

Now that you've pegged your faulty thinking, reframe the underlying assumption, and all its supportive thoughts, in a more positive light. Flip your thinking from focusing on negative emotions, faulty thinking, black or white thinking, cognitive distortions, and so on to focusing on any positive, measured thoughts that are closer to the truth. What could those negative thoughts look like when reframed?

_____

_____

_____

_____

_____

_____

_____

_____

_____

_____

_____

_____

_____

_____

_____

_____

_____

_____

Keep this method in mind as we progress so you can call upon it whenever you encounter negative thoughts or biases that will hamper your aging process.

KEY TAKEAWAYS FOR *GET A NEW ATTITUDE*

- Aging is often associated with health decline, cognitive decline, and depression, but research shows that many older adults maintain good health, cognitive function, and emotional well-being. Some become even more creative and focused. Aging can bring increased happiness, resilience, and mental strength.
- Despite common fears about aging, many people experience personal growth, emotional maturity, and increased happiness as they get older. Research shows happiness and mental health often improve in later life, with many older adults reporting greater life satisfaction than those in midlife.
- Most cognitive changes with age are mild, and older adults often maintain strong mental health, continue learning, and even excel in areas such as creativity and accumulated knowledge. Many people grow more satisfied with life and optimistic as they age, and dementia affects only a minority of elderly people.
- Cognitive reframing allows you to recognize and challenge unhelpful thought patterns so you can view situations from a more balanced and constructive perspective. By identifying distorted thoughts, questioning their validity, you can replace them with healthier alternatives and shift your mindset.

> "I've enjoyed every age I've been, and each has had its own individual merit. Every laugh line, every scar, is a badge I wear to show I've been present, the inner rings of my personal tree trunk that I display proudly for all to see. Nowadays, I don't want a "perfect" face and body; I want to wear the life I've lived."
>
> — PAT BENATAR, *BETWEEN A HEART AND A ROCK PLACE: A MEMOIR*

"Age has given me what I was looking for my entire life–it has given me *me*. It has provided time and experience and failures and triumphs and time-tested friends who have helped me step into the shape that was waiting for me. I fit into me now. I have an organic life, finally, not necessarily the one people imagined for me, or tried to get me to have. I have the life I longed for. I have become the woman I hardly dared imagine I would be."

— ANNE LAMOTT,
PLAN B: FURTHER THOUGHTS ON FAITH

Adjust
YOUR HABITS

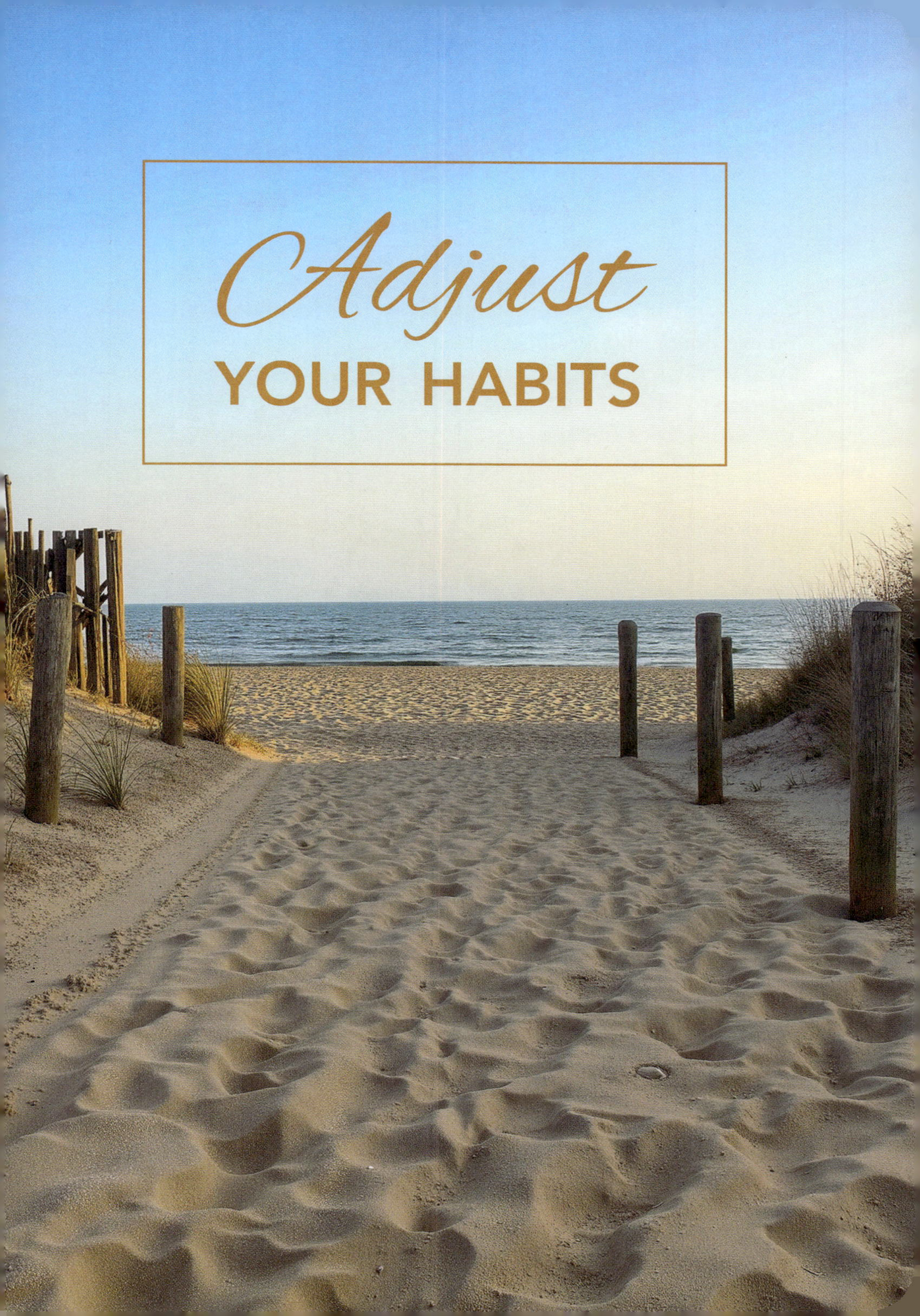

Adjust Your Habits

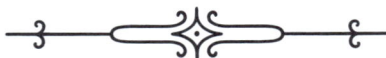

Now that you've adjusted your attitude, it's time to adjust your habits. The way you live now will undoubtedly have a monumental effect on how you age. If you've been making unhealthy choices, we want to help you turn them around to make the kinds of choices that will give you a leg up on aging gracefully. Let's begin by assessing where you are now.

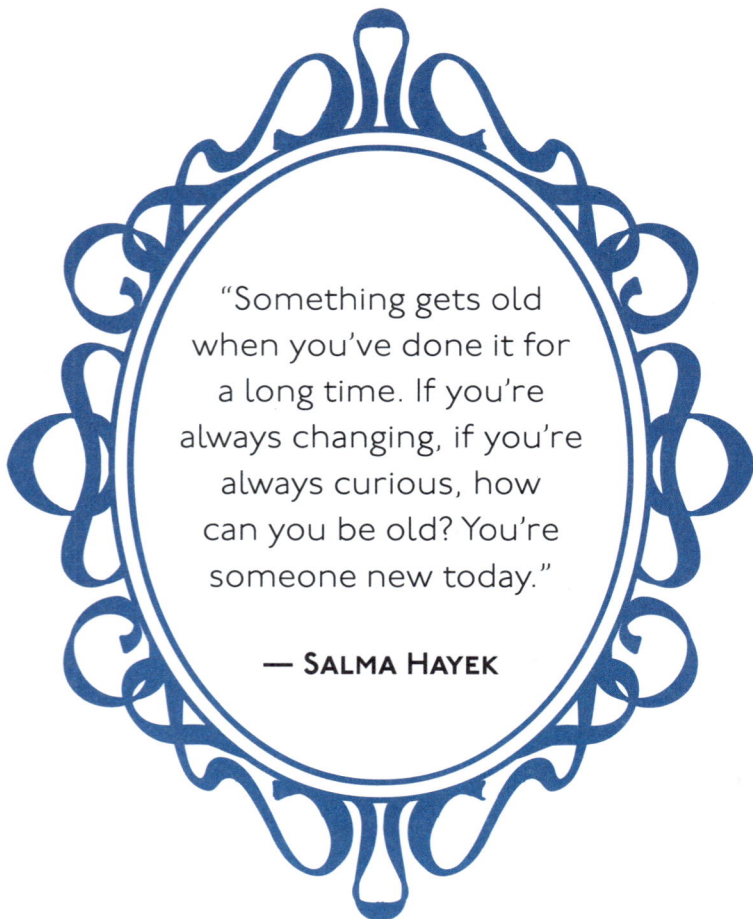

"Something gets old when you've done it for a long time. If you're always changing, if you're always curious, how can you be old? You're someone new today."

— **SALMA HAYEK**

ARE YOU IN THE BLUE ZONE?

A team of *National Geographic* researchers analyzed areas of the world where people lived longer and healthier than most of us (they focused on people who reached age 100 at a rate ten times higher than we do in the United States) and identified five areas that they called "blue zones" in which longevity is common. They then identified nine common-denominator attitudes and behaviors (dubbed the "power nine") that seemed to foster healthy aging.

1. **Move naturally.** The lifestyle of people in blue zones nudges them to move without thinking about it. They do their own housework and yardwork, for example.
2. **Find a purpose.** Having a sense of purpose added seven years to life expectancy.
3. **Downshift.** Superagers in blue zones actively reduced stress by pausing daily to rest, typically by thinking about their ancestors, praying, napping, and observing happy hour.
4. **Follow the 80 percent rule for eating.** Superagers stop eating when they feel 80 percent full, and they eat their smallest meal in the late afternoon or early evening and then don't eat again until the next morning.
5. **Follow a mostly plant-based diet.** These healthy agers eat a lot of beans and only eat meat about five times a month.
6. **Drink a moderate amount of alcohol.** Superagers limit themselves to one or two glasses per day, mostly of wine.*
7. **Be part of a faith-based community.** Over 90 percent of blue zone superagers belonged to a faith-based community.
8. **Focus on families.** Superagers put their families first, keep parents and grandparents close by, commit to their marriages, and heavily invest in their children.
9. **Maintain strong social networks.** Superagers belong to social groups that reinforce healthy behaviors. Most have a group of five friends who commit to each other for life.

*Note that more recent studies have found that drinking any alcohol is detrimental to your health and do not recommend even one glass of wine a night. It's the process of relaxing and reducing stress involved with enjoying a glass of wine that likely creates a positive effect anyway. Consider mocktails!

HOW'S YOUR POWER NINE?

Go through each of the "Power Nine" outlined on page 31 and identify how you're doing on each by highlighting **answers below that are closest to your reality.**

1. I physically move around a lot in my day-to-day life.
    I spend too much time sitting or watching TV.
    I make sure to get vigorous exercise at least three times a week.
    I lift weights to maintain muscle strength.

2. I have a sense of purpose that drives my life.
    I have a lifelong dream that I am pursuing.
    Beyond money or success, I have a driving force that motivates me.
    I am looking forward to the chance to reinvent myself when I retire.

3. I have stress-relief methods that I regularly use.
    I take time every day to downshift and relax.
    I often meditate or spend time being quiet and reflective.
    My life is balanced and satisfying.

4. I rarely overeat and tend to make healthier food choices.
    I eat too much processed or fatty foods.
    I overeat on a regular basis and always regret it.
    I should lose 20 percent of my weight.

5. I have cut back on the amount of red meat I eat.
    I like all types of meat and eat meat at almost every meal.
    I eat fish at least two times a week.
    I rarely eat vegetables or salad.

6. I am very conscious of limiting the amount of alcohol I drink.
   I love my cocktail hour and enjoy hard liquor more than two days a week.
   I often drink too much beer.
   I occasionally have a glass or two of wine with dinner.

7. I have a spiritual practice or community that is important to me.
   I was raised religious but rarely go to church anymore.
   I'm too busy to find a "special community."
   I don't feel a need to connect on a spiritual level.

8. I am close to and foster good relationships with my family.
   I like most of my family members but rarely spend time with them.
   Every time my family is gathered, we argue.
   I rarely talk to my extended family.

9. I value friendships and consistently make time to truly connect.
   I've had a small set of friends for years, but we rarely connect.
   I haven't made a new friend in ten years. Who has time?
   When I'm with friends, we keep our conversations surface level.

> "In spite of illness, in spite even of the archenemy sorrow, one can remain alive long past the usual date of disintegration if one is unafraid of change, insatiable in intellectual curiosity, interested in big things, and happy in small ways."
>
> — EDITH WHARTON

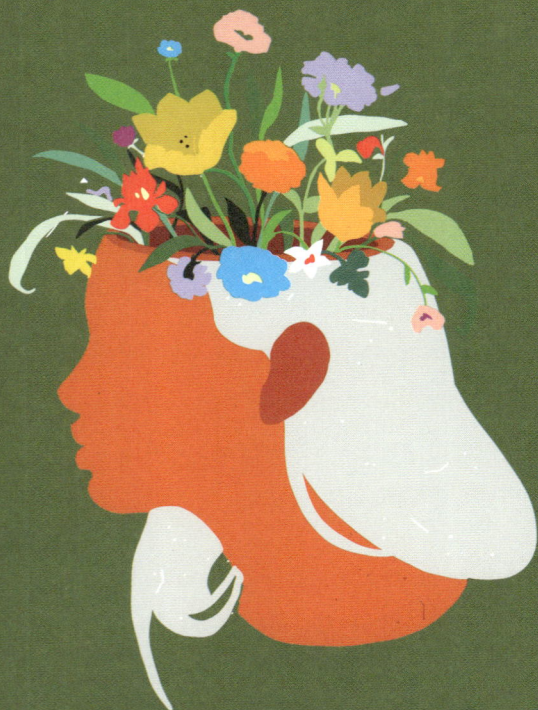

"There is a fountain of youth: it is your mind, your talents, the creativity you bring to your life and the lives of people you love. When you learn to tap this source, you will truly have defeated age."

— SOPHIA LOREN

How did you fare on your Power Nine? Did you identify areas you need to focus on and improve? What are they? Write each down along with ways you can alter or change those habits. Will you make a commitment to yourself to create goals that will help you work toward the healthiest choices?

_____
_____
_____
_____
_____
_____
_____
_____
_____
_____
_____
_____
_____
_____
_____
_____
_____
_____
_____
_____
_____
_____
_____

FOCUS ON POSITIVITY

Jane Fonda once told *Glamour* that she had a revelation when she approached age sixty. "I realized that I was approaching my third act—my final act—and that it wasn't a dress rehearsal. One of the things that I knew for sure is that I didn't want to get to the end with a lot of regrets, so how I lived up until the end was what was going to determine whether I had regrets." Fonda did a "life review" that helped her see things more clearly. "It totally changed the way I thought about myself and about how I wanted to live the last third of my life," she said. "And I realized the importance of being intentional about how we go through life."

Now in her eighties, Fonda said one of her biggest takeaways has been: "When you get older, you realize that staying healthy is joyful and critical because age isn't so much chronology. You can be very old at 84, which is my [current] age, but you can also be very young."

Jane was prescient in her approach. Research shows that people who view aging optimistically are more likely to engage in activities that support physical and mental health and social connection. In turn, these habits not only enhance longevity but also improve quality of life. It's never too late or too early to start planning for life's third act. If you take control of your narrative, maintain a positive attitude, and switch the lens, you can beautifully reframe your future.

If you think positively, you are also more likely to live longer. In a thirty-year study of sixty-three-year-old adults, the Yale School of Public Health found that elders who displayed an optimistic attitude lived another twenty-two years, while those who were pessimistic only lived another fifteen years. That's an extra seven years for optimists!

According to Katharine Esty, author of *Eighty Somethings,* how and when people think and speak about what they perceive as 'old age' is powerful. "People say, 'I'm older, I'm aging;' they'll use that phrasing, but not *'I'm old.'* If you have a positive attitude toward aging, you're going to live that (additional) 7.5 years longer."

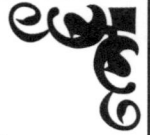

Have you done a 'life review' to review how you think about yourself and your regrets? Even if you have, take a moment now to write about your biggest regrets.

_____

_____

_____

_____

_____

_____

_____

_____

_____

What do these regrets reveal about your values, priorities, and future desires?

_____

_____

_____

_____

_____

_____

_____

How do you talk about your aging process? Do you view it positively, as in growing in wisdom and ability to focus more on family or fulfill ambitions, or do you tend to focus on unwelcome changes, like wrinkles or bodily aches and pains?

_____

_____

_____

_____

_____

_____

_____

_____

_____

_____

_____

_____

_____

_____

_____

_____

_____

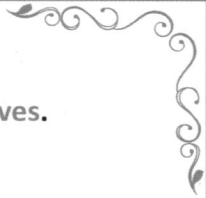

List five realities about aging that you will now see as positives.

1
_____

_____

_____

2
_____

_____

_____

3
_____

_____

_____

4
_____

_____

_____

5
_____

_____

_____

List five statements you could make about your own aging process and how you'll feel going forward that reflect a positive attitude.

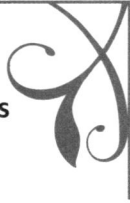

1 _____

_____

_____

2 _____

_____

_____

3 _____

_____

_____

4 _____

_____

_____

5 _____

_____

_____

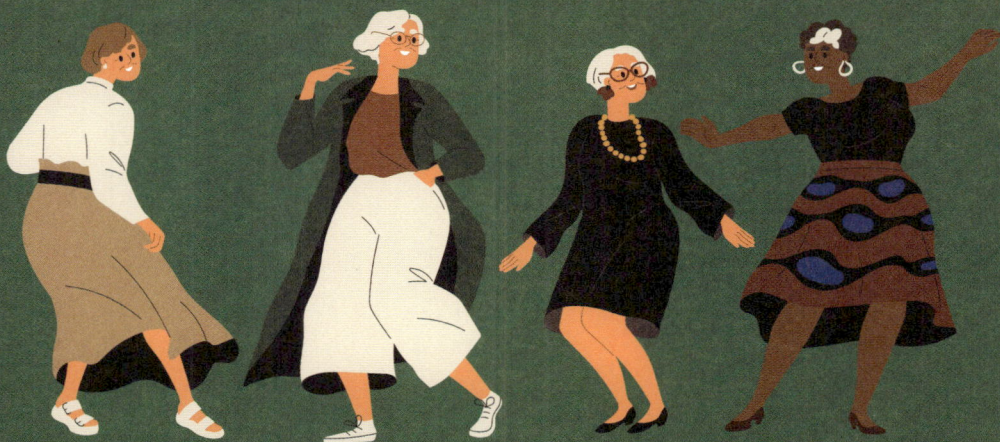

"Women have been brainwashed all our lives to hate our bodies. That's just the fact, and everything that surrounds us reminds us how imperfect we are, and everything is wrong with us . . . I'm not going to waste my passion, my energy, my curiosity, my money, and my life's purpose worrying about my body."

— EMMA THOMPSON

HOW POSITIVE ARE YOU?

One of the keys to a long, happy life is to focus on positivity, particularly about aging. The more you can flip negativity to positivity, the more doing so will become ingrained. So, let's see how well you're doing on positivity. Researchers coined the term "emodiversity" to describe a person's ability to possess a breath and abundance of positive emotions, such as:

Active	Curious	Joyful
Alert	Determined	Inspired
Amazed	Energetic	Interested
Amused	Engaged	Optimistic
At ease	Enthusiastic	Playful
Appreciation	Exuberant	Proud
Attentive	Excited	Relaxed
Calm	Generous	Self-assured
Cheerful	Grateful	Strong
Connected	Happy	Uplifted
	Invigorated	

Highlight the feelings on the previous page that you often experience. Which ones are a challenge? Why?

_____

_____

_____

_____

_____

_____

_____

_____

_____

_____

_____

_____

_____

_____

_____

_____

_____

_____

_____

_____

_____

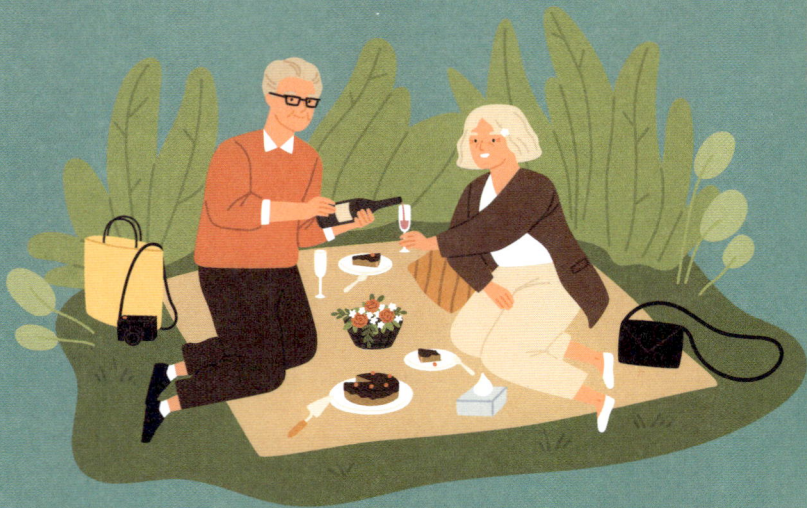

"People who take in more negative age beliefs tend to show worse physical, cognitive, and mental health. But the good news is that those who are exposed to or develop more positive age beliefs tend to show benefits in physical, cognitive, and mental health."

— BECCA LEVY,
BREAKING THE AGE CODE

Where in your life do you experience mostly happy feelings?

_____

_____

_____

_____

_____

_____

_____

_____

Where in your life do you feel the opposite? What erodes your positivity?

_____

_____

_____

_____

_____

_____

_____

_____

"Beautiful young people are accidents of nature,
but beautiful old people are works of art."

— ELEANOR ROOSEVELT

ARE YOU AN OPTIMIST OR A PESSIMIST?

We may be born with a disposition that leans one way or the other, or our life experiences may have greatly influenced whether we are optimistic or pessimistic. The point is that you can *reframe* the way you view situations to reflect a more positive, optimistic attitude.

What causes optimism in your life?

_____

_____

_____

What causes pessimism in your life?

_____

_____

_____

Which attitude do you feel most often, and why?

_____

_____

_____

"I am appalled that the term we use to talk about aging is 'anti.' Aging is as natural as a baby's softness and scent. Aging is human evolution in its pure form. Death, taxes, and aging."

— JAMIE LEE CURTIS

Think back to an experience that caused pessimism and see if you can find the positive in the situation. Write about the experience, focusing on the positive aspects you may have missed the first time around.

Some specific attitudes (mantras!) that will foster healthy aging include the following.

I will have more that I want to achieve.
I will have time to make serious and satisfying plans.
I will have enough resources to accomplish them.
I can and will succeed.
I want to continue growing and developing.
I want to keep working, volunteering, mentoring, and being social
I want to continue being influential and important.
By being proactive and staying on top of things, I can live a lot longer.

Pause to write your own list of positive thoughts (strive for ten!). Once you've created those positive thoughts speak or write them often as affirmations that will reinforce your determination to live a healthy, happy, productive, and fulfilling old age. The more you reinforce those positive thoughts, the more they'll help you going forward.

1 _____

_____

_____

2 _____

_____

_____

3 _____

_____

_____

4 _____

_____

_____

5

6

7

8

9

10

> "When I turned sixty, I looked in the mirror and I said, 'Denzel, this is not a dress rehearsal. This is life'."
>
> **— DENZEL WASHINGTON**

HOW TO LEARN OPTIMISM

Even if you don't tend towards optimism, there's sufficient time to change your attitude. Dr. Martin Seligman, author of *Learned Optimism*, theorized that a positive attitude could be learned and developed. He explained by delineating what he calls the "ABC response to adversity":

A. Adversity happens
B. A belief is formed
C. Consequences, actions, and associated feelings occur.

Later he added D and E, steps designed to further develop positive thinking.

D. Disputation or consciously generating counter evidence to dispute and release the belief
E. Energization, noticing how your mood and the outcome changes because of working through ABCD.

It's as simple as this: The more you learn to objectively view situations, flip pessimism to optimism, and reinforce the process, the easier your aging process will be.

> "It's almost as if we have failed if we don't remain 25 for the rest of our lives. Like it's a personal failure. Like it's our fault that at 40 years old, I don't still look like I'm 25. 'Oh, I'm sorry. I apologize I wasn't able to defy nature… I feel that aging is a privilege. It's something that I feel very honored that I get to do."
>
> — **CAMERON DIAZ**

Think of the time when something happened that pitched you into despair. Using Dr. Seligman's ABCDE method, work through the memory:

What happened?

_____

_____

What did you believe about what happened? Which beliefs caused or reinforced negativity or pessimism?

_____

_____

What did you feel and do because of the experience and your reaction to it?

_____

_____

How could you counteract the belief(s) that led to feeling disillusionment and negativity?

_____

_____

How do you feel once you embrace the counterargument and see the experience in a new light?

_____

_____

KEEP A GRATITUDE JOURNAL

Focusing far more on positive, uplifting thoughts counteracts a lapse into negative thoughts and fosters positivity. Do you celebrate the good? What are you grateful to have in your life? At work? Writing down three pleasant surprises you experience each day will train you to focus more on positive happenings in your life. If you don't like writing in a journal each night, apps like Day One, Gratitude Plus, and Flavors of Gratefulness may be your cup of tea.

Write down at least three things you feel particularly grateful for and why.

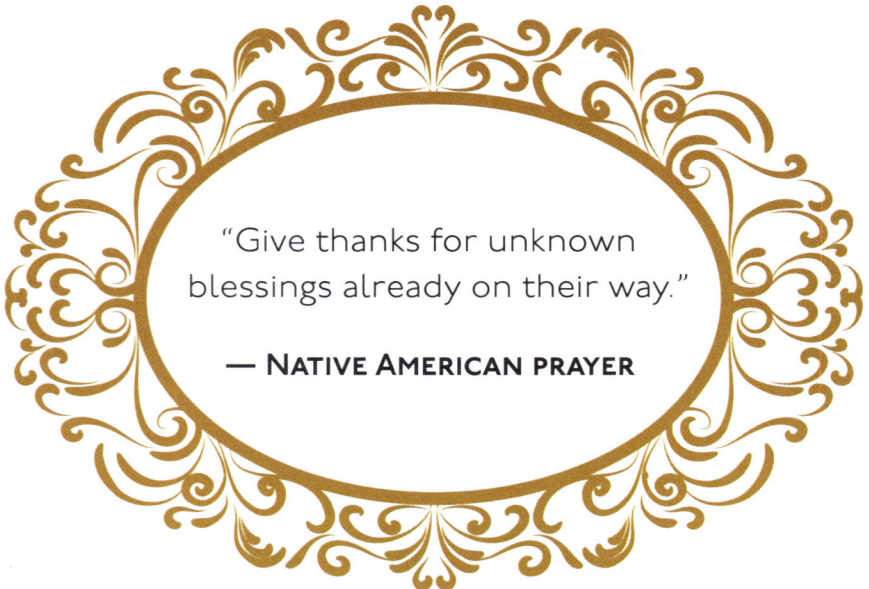

_____

_____

_____

_____

_____

_____

_____

"Give thanks for unknown
blessings already on their way."

— NATIVE AMERICAN PRAYER

USE A GRATITUDE JAR

If you don't want to write in a gratitude journal each night, you can try a 'gratitude jar.' Simply write down one thing you're grateful for each day and drop the slip of paper into the designated jar. Once a month, or so, you can pull out a handful of slips, then revisit and celebrate the many good things that happened in your life.

What are you grateful for in regard to your health? Your job? Your family? Your friends?

_____

_____

_____

_____

What kind of experiences fill your heart with gratitude?

_____

_____

_____

_____

FAKING IT IS OKAY

If you don't typically feel optimistic, it may prove helpful to simply pretend *that you do. Try simply acting* as if *you feel positive and optimistic in any given situation. In doing so, you may find your viewpoint really has flipped from anxiety, fear, and negativity to enthusiastic, energized, trusting, and hopeful.*

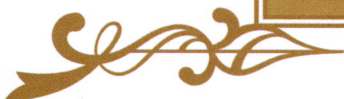

FOCUS ON GROWTH

In an October 2024 *Psychologytoday.com* blog posting about ageism, Sam Carr, PhD, a social scientist and researcher, reported that, as people age, they are susceptible to existential tiredness. He proposes that this results from no desire for, or mourning of, a future; only a profound sense that the journey is over yet drags on painfully and indefinitely. Fortunately, he suggests a solution: "Finding growth and unexpected gains in old age may help combat existential tiredness," Carr said.

This suggests that existential weariness can be remedied by *reframing* old age as a time for growth, rather than the end of growth, and then providing opportunities for that growth via part-time work, art, music, creative writing classes, or volunteer jobs, to name a few possibilities.

Most of us get locked into work schedules and lifestyles that are so demanding we rarely have time to explore new avenues or even think about expanding our world. As you age, however, it is vital to look for opportunities to grow—mentally, physically, socially, and spiritually. This requires you to pay attention to how you're living your life now and to seriously contemplate how you want to be living in the next phase of life.

Those who focus on growing as they age stay younger because:

1. They are stimulated by newness: their brains both create new neurons and keep the older ones firing. Their minds stay more alert and sharper.

2. They discover and embrace new activities that tend to keep them physically active.

3. Being 'out there' in the world helps them discover new passions and make new friends.

"Today I am 65 years old. I still look good. I appreciate and enjoy my age. A lot of people resist transition and therefore never allow themselves to enjoy who they are. Embrace the change, no matter what it is; once you do, you can learn about the new world you're in and take advantage of it. You still bring to bear all your prior experience, but you are riding on another level. It's completely liberating."

— NIKKI GIOVANNI

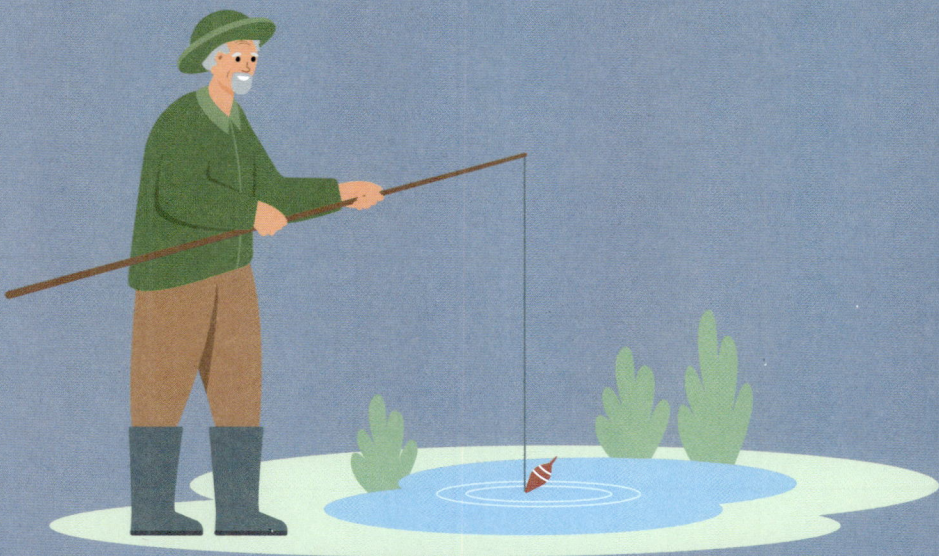

REVIEW YOUR CURRENT LIFESTYLE

How many hours do you spend working?

Commuting?

Worrying about work?

_____

_____

_____

_____

_____

_____

_____

_____

Does your work schedule permit time for outside interests or leisure activities? What do you do with that time?

_____

_____

_____

_____

_____

_____

_____

_____

Are you doing what you'd most like to be doing? If not, why not? How could you change this?

_____

_____

_____

_____

_____

_____

_____

_____

_____

_____

_____

_____

"Growing older gracefully means having a keen curiosity about learning things about the world that you didn't know yesterday, no matter how many yesterdays you've had."

— PADMA LAKSHMI

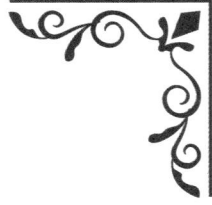

What's been missing in your life? If you could do *anything*, what would you do?

_____

_____

_____

_____

_____

_____

_____

_____

Do you foresee growth opportunities as you age? Are there specific areas in which you'd like to grow?

_____

_____

_____

_____

_____

_____

_____

_____

STILL WORKING

According to the U.S. Bureau of Labor Statistics, the number of workers sixty-five and older has mushroomed by 117 percent in a span of the last twenty years. Remarkably, the employment of individuals seventy-five and older has increased by the same percentage.

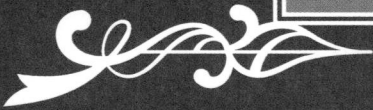

"How do we continue to challenge ourselves, to interest ourselves, learn new things, be more helpful to other people, be the person that your friends and family need or want? How do we continue to evolve? How do we navigate life to have even deeper experiences? That's what aging should be about."

— JULIANNE MOORE

BUILD RESILIENCE

According to Jeannette Guerrasio, MD, author of *Embrace Aging*, resilience is "the ability to recover from difficult experiences, setbacks, and tragedies and to be able to move forward, learn, adapt, and grow from one's challenges." Resilience, she says, can be learned from exposure to a series of very challenging but manageable experiences of increasing difficulty and cites her experience as a resident as an example. Each day would bring massive challenges but, once she'd successfully met them, the next day she'd feel stronger.

Because it comes with ongoing changes, challenges, setbacks, and obstacles, successful aging will require massive resiliency, which comes from growth. How you address challenges, the choices you make daily in how you live your life create or erode resilience. Let's discuss maladaptive behaviors versus adaptive behaviors that either erode or create resilience.

Dr. Guerrasio created a list of what she calls adaptive versus maladaptive behaviors.

In reviewing the list on the following page, highlight your strengths in one color and the areas where you need improvement in another color. How do you measure up at this point? Where are you falling short? What do you most need to work on?

_____

_____

_____

_____

_____

_____

_____

_____

Adaptive Behaviors

Confronting problems directly and realistically

Recognizing and changing unhealthy emotional reactions

Practicing mindfulness

Nurturing and protecting your body

Creating and following a moral compass

Maintaining cognitive and emotional flexibility

Fostering self-compassion

Strengthening optimism (positive reframing), humor

Seeking and accepting help

Being empathetic towards others

Maladaptive Behaviors

Escaping problems, denial, avoidance

Succumbing to feelings of distress

Not addressing anxiety

Blaming others, venting

Excessive risk-taking behaviors

Lying to others and yourself

Allowing fear to stop you

Ruminating and persevering

Dwelling on the negative

Failing to address physical symptoms

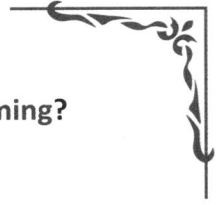

Are there certain challenges in your life that feel overwhelming?
How do you respond to these challenges?

_____

_____

_____

_____

_____

How could you reframe the way you view that type of challenge?

_____

_____

_____

_____

How could you address it with a healthier, more resilient mindset?

_____

_____

_____

_____

_____

Are you **flexible** or **fixed** in your temperament? Thoughts? Behavior? Responses? Is there one aspect of your life that finds you in the maladaptive category more than the adaptive one?

_____

_____

_____

_____

Do you offer yourself **compassion** for perceived mistakes? If not, why? In which instances do you most harshly judge yourself?

_____

_____

_____

_____

"I'm never going to be able to look like X, Y, and Z, especially as I become 50, 55; 60. So it's like: how do I feel? How am I holding myself? Do I like myself? What is my anxiety level? Am I strong? Yeah, I'm bummed that, for some reason, at 51, it's like all the elasticity's going. But if I look at a 28-year-old model on Instagram and think my stomach's supposed to look like that, I'll just go into a depression. So, I've really tried to divorce myself from that comparison."

— GWYNETH PATROW

CREATE A BENCHMARK FOR YOUR RESILIENCE

Life's challenges foster and build resilience. Recognizing all the challenges you've overcome provides a great benchmark for going forward. Reinforcing how well you've done in the past and giving yourself both recognition and credit for your victories will inspire you to meet new challenges with enthusiasm and grit. Identifying any weaknesses that forestalled success can help you beef up the areas where you've fallen short in the past.

Make a list of ten challenges you've faced and briefly note how you overcame them.

1 _____

_____

2 _____

_____

3 _____

_____

4 _____

_____

5 _____

_____

6 _____

_____

7

8

9

10

What strengths did you bring to the challenges?

What did you learn about yourself and your abilities?

"At thirty, I used to exercise to look good. At the age of fifty to be fit, and at seventy not to be padded in a bed. At eighty, to be able to live without assistance. Now, at ninety-nine, I do it out of pure defiance."

— DICK VAN DYKE

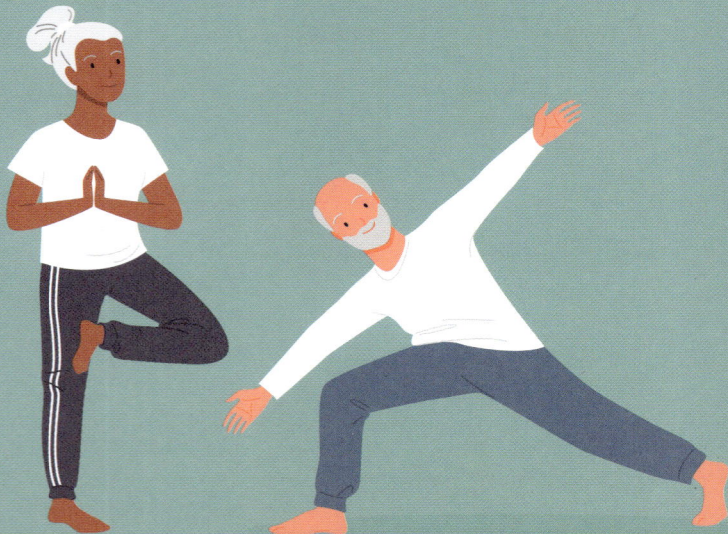

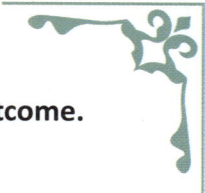

Think back to challenges that didn't produce the desired outcome. What went wrong? Was there something you failed to do?

_____

_____

_____

_____

_____

Did these less-than-successful challenges reveal something about yourself that you need to bolster going forward?

_____

_____

_____

_____

_____

_____

What specific steps could you take to develop greater resilience?

_____

_____

_____

_____

_____

_____

BOLSTERING RESILIENCE

When it comes to aging gracefully, resilience extends far beyond enduring adversity; resilience is the strength and confidence you develop over time to thrive in its aftermath. Much like a tree deepens its roots in response to trauma, think of resilience as the strategies you've used to conquer challenges and deepen your understanding of life. Resilience is the personal *chutzpah* that helps you adapt to change, effectively cope with health challenges, maintain a sense of hopefulness, and develop robust coping skills, such as stress management techniques. There are specific things you can do to bolster your resilience now and while aging gracefully. For example:

- View any perceived weaknesses or challenges simply as areas where improvement is needed; rather than berating yourself, use your faculties, knowledge, and creativity to come up with ways to grow within those experiences.
- Don't let being afraid to fail keep you from taking creative and social risks; view perceived 'mistakes' as opportunities to develop greater resilience.
- Take up a worthy cause to improve flexibility, thinking, empathy, and purpose. The more you look 'outward' rather than 'inward,' the stronger you become.
- Take advantage of opportunities to learn something new, which will stimulate your mind, increase flexibility, and help you refocus your attention when needed.
- Record your experiences, your responses, and your emotions in a journal; use the entries as a springboard for growth and a way to give yourself credit for progress and thereby reinforce your burgeoning resilience.

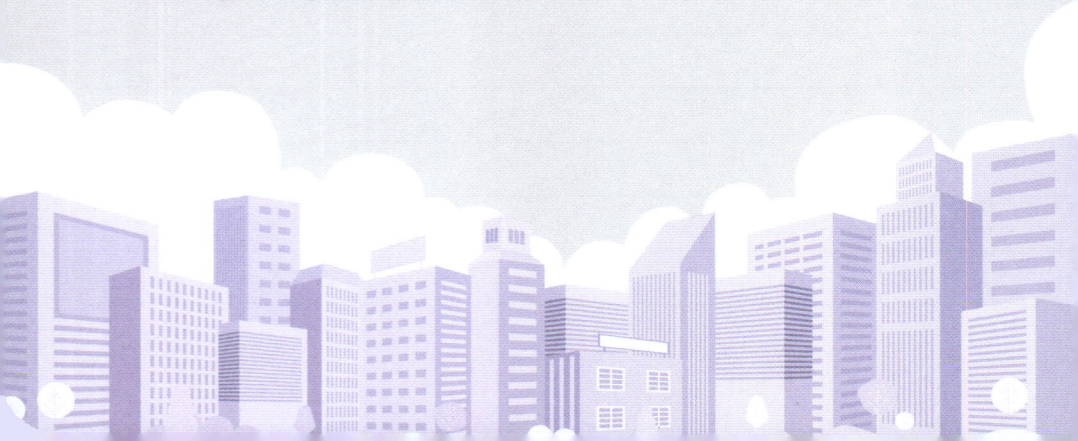

Make a list of your skills and strengths. Give yourself credit for as many as you can.

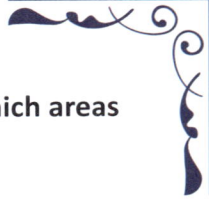

Taking an **honest look** at your current level of resilience, which areas do you see as the weakest?

_____

_____

_____

_____

_____

What **worthy cause** are you willing to take on?

_____

_____

_____

_____

_____

What would be something **new** and **challenging** that you could commit to learning?

_____

_____

_____

_____

_____

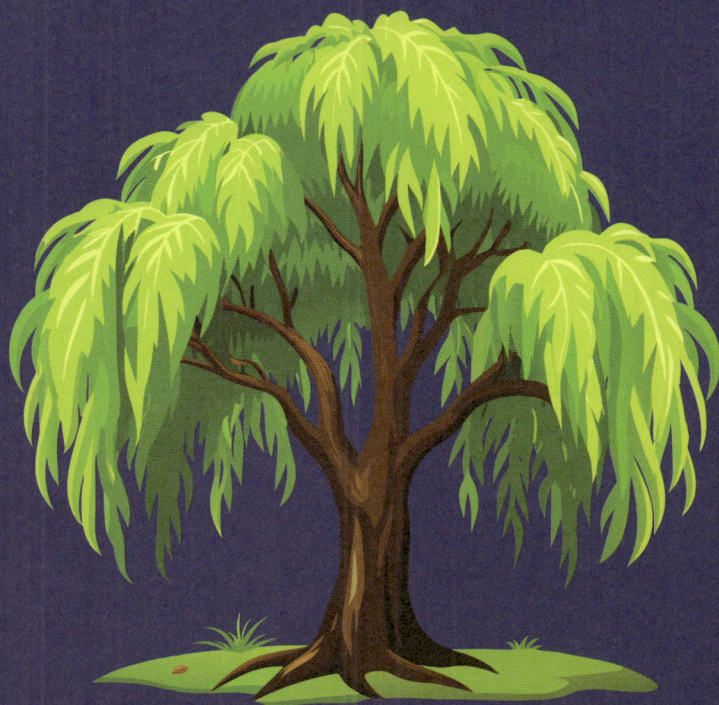

"Notice that the stiffest tree is most easily cracked, while the bamboo or willow survives by bending with the wind."

— BRUCE LEE

BOLSTER YOUR COURAGE

You've likely heard the adage: growing old is not for sissies. It's a popular adage because it's true, particularly as you age into your eighties. The challenges you must face grow over time, and those who face them with courage fare the best. Here are six aspects of life that reflect areas in which you'll need courage and effective ways to bolster your courage:

1. **Physical:** Move forward with resiliency, balance, and awareness.
2. **Social:** Be fully and unapologetically yourself.
3. **Moral:** Do what you know is morally right, regardless of situation.
4. **Emotional:** Feel, acknowledge, and release all your emotions, sans guilt or attachment.
5. **Intellectual:** Learn, unlearn, and relearn with an eager, open, and flexible mind.
6. **Spiritual:** Live with purpose and meaning, while employing a heart-centered approach towards all life and oneself.

In which areas listed above are you most courageous?

_____

_____

_____

_____

_____

In which areas do you need to grow?

_____

_____

_____

_____

_____

What will you commit to doing that will foster courage going forward?

_____

_____

_____

_____

_____

_____

_____

_____

_____

_____

_____

_____

_____

DON'T LET THE OLD MAN IN

While they were golfing together one day, the late country music artist Toby Keith asked Clint Eastwood his secret to a vibrant old age. Eastwood replied, "I just get up every morning and go out. And I don't let the old man in." Inspired by this conversation, Toby Keith then wrote the song, "Don't Let the Old Man In," which became the theme song of Clint's movie, The Mule.

ADOPT A GROWTH MINDSET

People with fixed mindsets view mistakes and challenges as a sign of their own incompetence and tend to give up. They view themselves as failures and thus stop trying. Those who develop a growth mindset view setbacks as chances to learn and opportunities for growth. They don't fault themselves; they learn from their mistakes and use that knowledge to seek a new pathway. Those who experienced high-quality, loving relationships as children—and in their current lives—often develop a growth mindset.

Did you feel loved as a small child?

Did you feel safe and supported as a small child?

Did you see your parents endure challenges and come out the other end?

Did you experience any traumas that may have hampered a sense of security and safety?

If any of the above were true for you, write any thoughts you have on how they have affected your ability to embrace change throughout your life.

_____

_____

_____

_____

_____

_____

If you weren't sufficiently loved and supported as a child, or didn't see productive behaviors modeled, you may be unconsciously holding yourself back and need to focus more than others on developing a growth mindset. The way you do that is to embrace efforts to expand your world, open to new experiences, and make learning new skills or hobbies a priority. The growth mindset is all about _expansion_ as a strategy for staying alert, focused, invigorated, motivated, and engaged. A growth mindset benefits your brain in a multitude of ways that will bolster and support your ability to age gracefully.

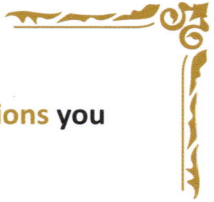

How could you commit to growing right now? List three actions you will take to grow.

1

_____

_____

_____

_____

_____

2

_____

_____

_____

_____

_____

3

_____

_____

_____

_____

_____

JUST SAY 'YES'

As we age, many of us shy away from doing or trying new things. Whether we just get too lazy or set in our ways or experience anxiety when new ideas are offered, our first reaction to invitations and opportunities outside our comfort zone is to say 'no,' but doing so limits opportunities to grow.

Instead of habitually anticipating a negative outcome and thereby turning down opportunities, practice just saying 'yes.' If someone wants you to go to an exotic restaurant and you're afraid you won't like the food, just say 'yes' anyway. You may have a pleasant surprise, and even if you don't like the food, you might enjoy the ambiance and company. At the very least, you'd have a new story to tell your best friend. If someone wants to try a new sport, even if you're afraid you'll look incompetent or foolish, just say 'yes' and embrace it to your full capacity. You may discover a new, and very healthy, obsession.

Growing is about expanding and learning new things, throughout life. If you always just say 'no,' you are denying yourself opportunities to experience the kind of lifelong learning that invigorates the brain. New experiences create new neurons and new neuronal pathways, both of which keep your brain active and thereby improve overall brain functioning.

What are three activities or experiences you would typically decline that you could choose to try?

1 _____

_____

2 _____

_____

3 _____

_____

Look for places or situations or experiences that have become too entrenched or habitual and break that boredom, even if it requires doing the opposite of what you'd normally do. The next time you go out for a walk, try walking in the opposite direction than you normally do; try reading outside during the day when you normally read in bed at night; try reaching out to someone you haven't talked to in a long time when it's long been more typical of you to rarely do so. Seek novelty and you'll encourage beneficial growth.

How often do you do something fear-inducing or, at the very least, novel? What are you willing to do to foster change?

_____

_____

_____

_____

_____

_____

_____

_____

_____

_____

_____

_____

_____

_____

_____

_____

- People in long-lived cultures incorporate movement into daily life, have a strong sense of purpose, and manage stress through restful rituals such as prayer and napping. They follow healthy eating habits—stopping before full, favoring plant-based diets, and drinking alcohol moderately. Strong social ties, faith-based communities, and deep family connections also play key roles in supporting their well-being and longevity.

- Research has found that those who view aging positively tend to stay healthier, live longer, and enjoy a better quality of life, gaining up to seven more years simply through an optimistic mindset.

- Those who prioritize growth as they age remain more youthful because engaging in new experiences keeps their minds sharp, their bodies active, and their social lives enriched. Reframing aging as a time for exploration and development helps you to discover renewed purpose and vitality.

- Resilience in aging isn't just about surviving hardships—it's about building the strength, confidence, and adaptability to grow from them and thrive. You can bolster resilience by embracing challenges as opportunities for growth, taking creative and social risks, engaging in purposeful causes, learning new things, and reflecting through journaling to recognize and reinforce your progress.

- As we age, it's easy to fall into the habit of saying 'no' to new experiences out of fear, discomfort, or routine—but doing so limits personal growth and brain vitality. Saying 'yes' more often opens the door to unexpected joys, strengthens social connections, and stimulates brain health by creating new neural pathways and keeping the mind engaged.

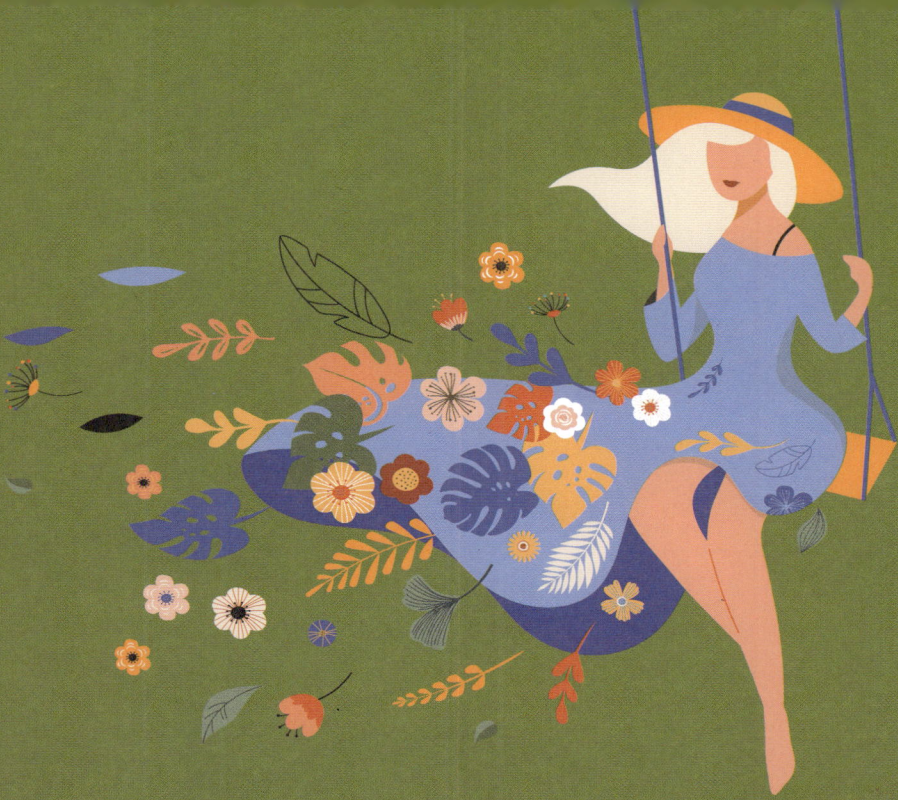

"I find myself thinking about being youthful and timeless at every age. At some point aging is going to happen, but until then, you decide how strong you're going to be. How much you're going to move. How much you're going to work. How active you are going to be in your mind, with your life, with your body. You decide. And you can keep it strong. You can keep it good."

— JENNIFER LOPEZ

"There's so much misogynist chatter in response to the *Sex and the City* reboot *And Just Like That*. Especially on social media. Everyone has something to say. 'She has too many wrinkles, she doesn't have enough wrinkles.' It almost feels as if people don't want us to be perfectly okay with where we are, as if they almost enjoy us being pained by who we are today, whether we choose to age naturally and not look perfect, or whether you do something if that makes you feel better. I know what I look like. I have no choice. What am I going to do about it? Stop aging? Disappear?"

— SARAH JESSICA PARKER

Nourish
YOUR BODY
AND BRAIN

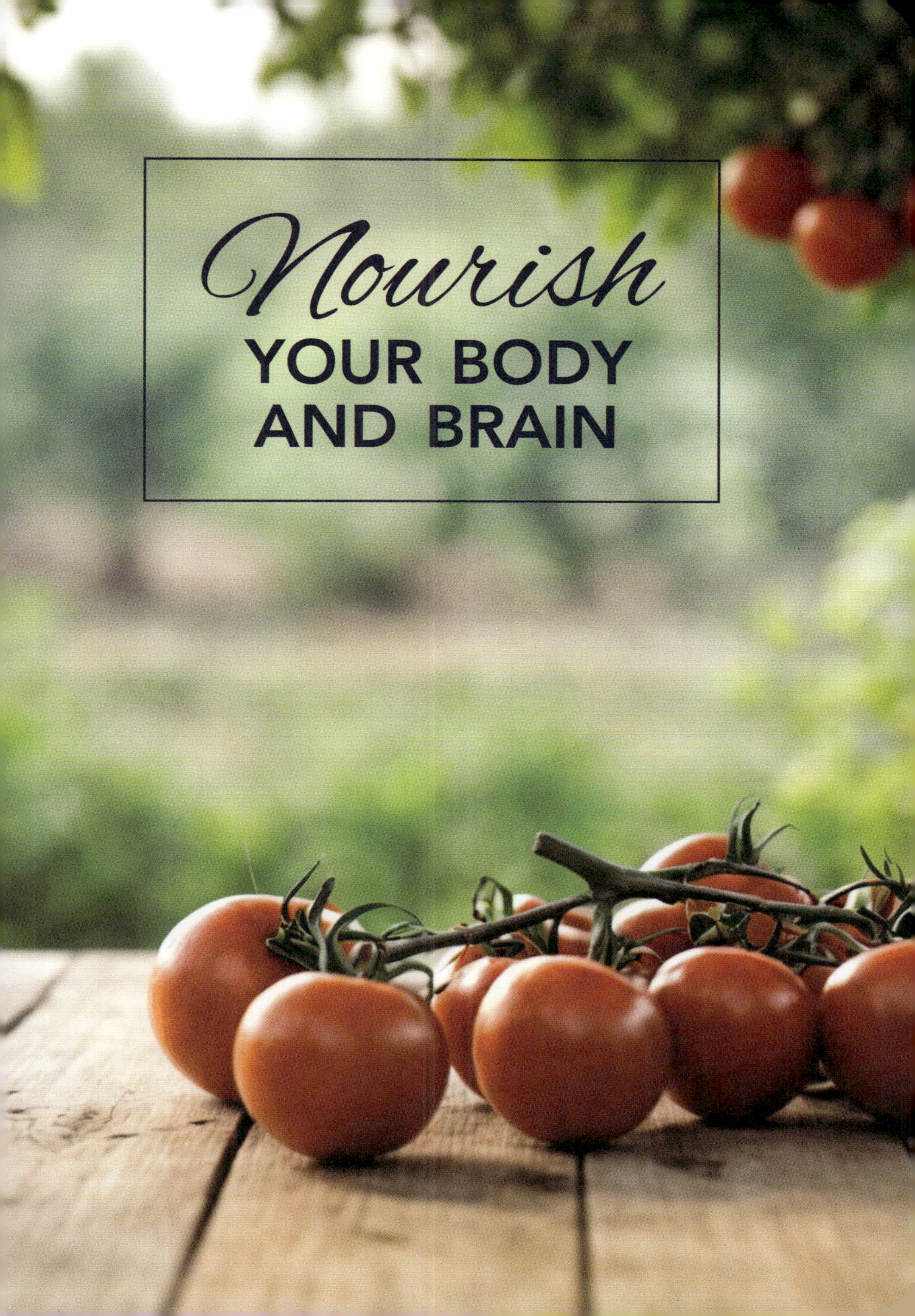

Nourish Your Body and Brain

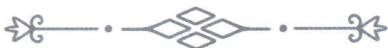

Without question, your body and brain are going to go through changes. No one has successfully created a 'youth serum' that will significantly delay the aging process. Your body and brain will lose ground, but how much ground can be greatly affected by how diligently you work to nourish your body and brain now, and as you age gracefully.

MAKE GOOD CHOICES

As your body and brain change, it's helpful to focus on all the power, strength, clarity, and function you still have. Yes, you'll see declines in strength, ability, and energy—and later memory—but rather than focus on the negative aspects, focus on what remains good. Keep your eye on the prize: You will still be alive, still healthy, still highly functioning, still capable of change, and ripe for a new adventure.

What you need to do will change over time, but there are essentials to maintaining good health that should rightfully either start or ramp up in middle age. Of course, the more you do to bolster your health and the longer you sustain those healthy new habits, the easier growing older will proceed. However, if you do only the following, you're still setting the stage for a healthier and happier old age:

- Choose your food carefully
- Regularly sleep well
- Stay physically active
- Keep your brain at peak capacity
- Boost your energy.

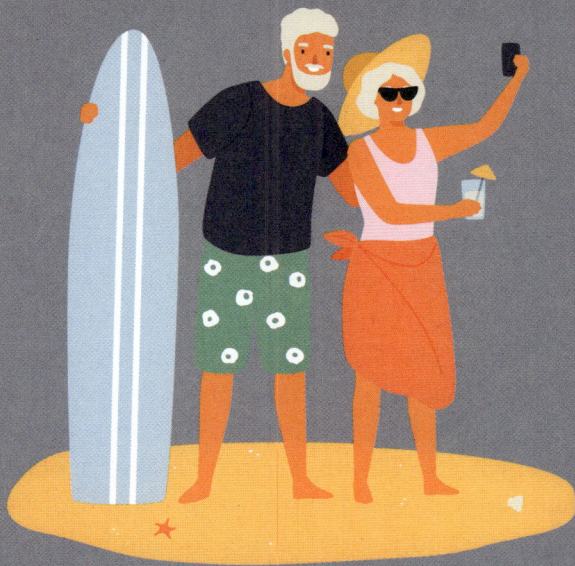

"I just don't think of age and time in respect of years. I just have too much experience of people in their 70s who are vigorous and useful and people that are 35 that are in [lousy] physical shape and can't think straight. I don't think age has that much to do with it."

— HARRISON FORD

IMPROVE YOUR DIET

'Genetics load the gun, and lifestyle pulls the trigger': that's a common expression about the effects of aging. In an article published in *Medical News Today*, Dr. Sheryl Ross used the expression, adding "Harmful, and avoidable, lifestyle habits include smoking, inactivity, eating an unhealthy diet (too many saturated fats, refined carbohydrates, highly processed and fast food!), excessive alcohol consumption, and not sleeping well individually and collectively contribute to heart disease, high blood pressure, high cholesterol, certain cancers, and cognitive decline."

Scientists define a healthy ager as someone who reaches the age of seventy without experiencing a major chronic condition, and who also maintains good cognitive, physical, and mental health. A 30-year study on optimal dietary patterns that followed the eating habits of more than 100,000 middle-aged adults (aged 39-69) found that what you eat in your thirties, forties, and fifties affects your health in your seventies. The study revealed that the adults who adhered most closely to diets rich in pant-based foods and ate fewer ultra-processed foods had a far higher likelihood of aging beyond seventy with-out experiencing a major chronic disease. Specifically, the adults who fared best adhered to a diet that limited processed foods and rather included consuming high amounts of fruits, vegetables, whole grains, unsaturated fats, nuts, and beans.

They found that a healthy ager needs to work towards a high HEI (Healthy Eating Index) score which means a diet focused on eating:

- 5 servings per day of vegetables
- 1 *extra serving* of green leafy vegetables
- 4 -5 servings of fruit per day
- 5-6 servings of whole grains
- 1 serving per day of a plant protein: nuts or legumes
- 1 serving of fish per week
- Using plant oils as your main culinary fat.

The study found that the participants who most closely followed an HEI pattern of eating had an 86 percent higher chance of healthy aging at age seventy and a 2.2 times higher likelihood of healthy aging at seventy-five.

Optimal dietary patterns for healthy aging. Tessier, A., Wang, F., Korat, A.A., Eliassen, A.H., Chavarro, J., Grodstein, F., Li, J., Liang, L., Willett, W.C., Sun, Q., Stampfer, M.J., Hu, F.B., Guasch-Ferré, M. *Nature Medicine* (2025). DOI: 10.1038/s41591-025-03570-5, https://www.nature.com/articles/s41591-025-03570-5

TRY THE 80 PERCENT RULE

In Japan, many practice "Hara Hachi Bu," a form of mindful eating focused on moderation. Those who follow this practice eat until they are 80 percent full and then stop. This is believed to help you maintain energy throughout the day. It also seems to help you to maintain a healthier weight.

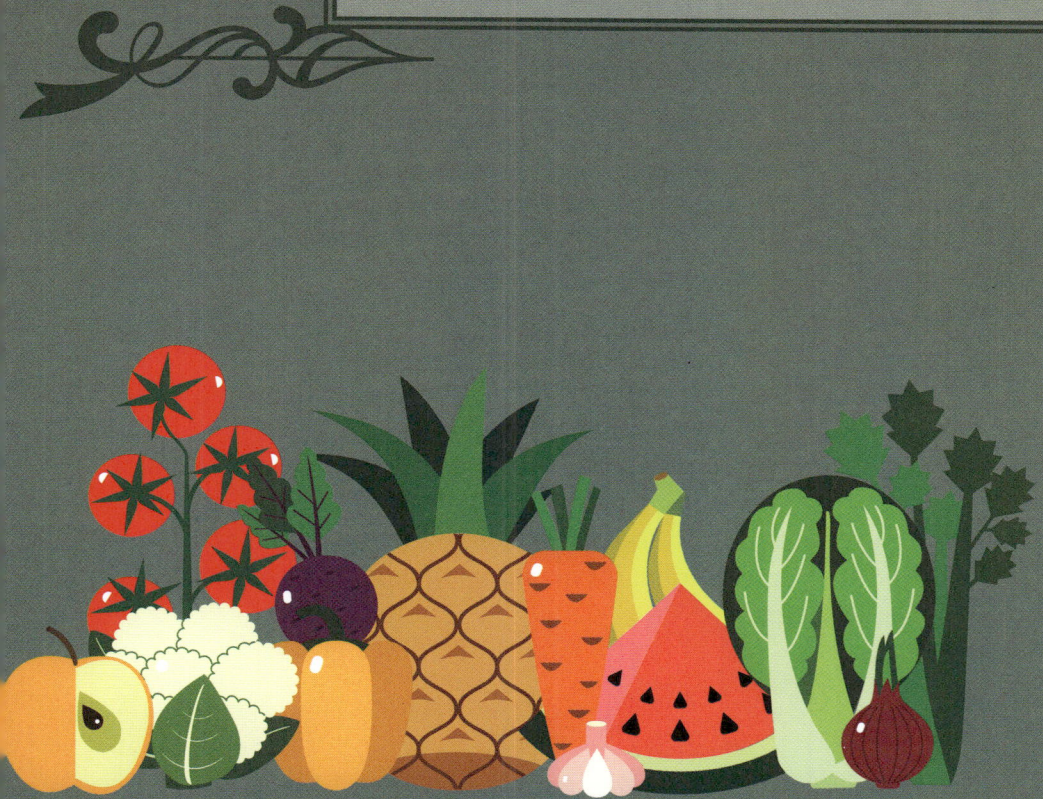

KEY NUTRIENTS AND FOODS FOR HEALTHY AGING

Beyond general healthy eating, specific nutrients and food groups play targeted roles in supporting age-specific health needs:

- ✓ **Calcium and Vitamin D** are vital for bone health; aim for 1,000-1,200 mg of calcium and 600-800 IU of vitamin D daily. Sources include dairy products, fortified plant-based beverages, tofu, canned salmon with bones, dark green vegetables, and egg yolks.

- ✓ **Unsaturated Fats**, found in fatty fish such as salmon, nuts, seeds, avocados, and olive oil, contribute to heart health, reduce inflammation, and protect against oxidative damage.

- ✓ **Extra virgin olive oil**, rich in monounsaturated fats and antioxidants, has been linked to a lower risk of chronic diseases and may even reduce severe skin aging due to its strong anti-inflammatory properties.

- ✓ **Antioxidants**, abundant in colorful fruits and vegetables, green tea, and nuts, combat free radicals, unstable molecules that can damage cells and accelerate aging. Green tea, specifically, is high in polyphenols that may reduce the risk of heart disease, neurological decline, and premature aging.

- ✓ **Fiber**, both soluble and insoluble, is crucial for digestive health, blood sugar management, and maintaining a healthy weight. It is found in oats, barley, beans, lentils, fruits, vegetables, and whole grains.

- ✓ **Lean Proteins** from sources like beans, lentils, tofu, lean meats, fish, and eggs are essential for maintaining muscle mass and overall bodily function.

How are you doing at maximizing your Healthy Eating Index (HEI)? Where are you falling short?

_____

_____

_____

_____

What will you choose to add or bolster going forward?

_____

_____

_____

_____

Where are you falling short on key nutrients and foods?

_____

_____

_____

_____

How can you change the way you eat to incorporate more HEI foods and nutrients into your daily diet?

_____

_____

_____

_____

WHAT NOT TO EAT

What you avoid or limit is as important as what you eat. Excessive consumption of certain food categories significantly increases the risk of chronic conditions that impede healthy aging. These include:

- **Processed foods high in sodium**: These contribute to high blood pressure, heart disease, and type 2 diabetes. Reducing salt intake and flavoring foods with herbs and spices is advisable.

- **Added sugars and sugary beverages:** High sugar intake is linked to type 2 diabetes and other chronic conditions.

- **Saturated and trans fats:** Found in fatty meats, processed meats, high-fat dairy, and deep-fried foods, these increase the risk of heart disease.

- **Red and processed meats:** Long-term studies have shown an inverse association between high intake of these and healthy aging outcomes.

- **Alcohol:** Excessive consumption can negatively impact bone mass and overall health. More recent studies found that drinking any alcohol can be detrimental.

Because chronic diseases such as heart disease, type 2 diabetes, and hypertension are major factors that compromise quality of life and independence in later years, actively limiting these detrimental food categories becomes a powerful strategy to stay healthy and maintain vitality.

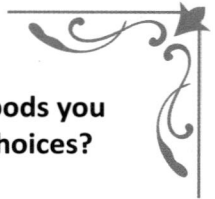

Identify any problem foods in your typical diet. Are these foods you can severely limit? What's a strategy for making healthier choices?

_____

_____

_____

_____

_____

_____

_____

_____

_____

From the list of undesirable choices, which ones do you need to address? What's the strategy for making sure you eat less of those foods and more of the desirable foods?

_____

_____

_____

_____

_____

_____

_____

_____

_____

IMPROVE YOUR SLEEP HABITS

According to the National Library of Medicine, recent studies demonstrate known and suspected relationships between inadequate sleep and a wide range of disorders, including hypertension, obesity and type 2 diabetes, impaired immune functioning, cardiovascular disease and arrhythmia, mood disorders, neurodegeneration and dementia, and even loneliness.

A recent study published in the *BMC Public Health Journal* explored how different sleep duration patterns relate to 'successful aging' among older adults. The study emphasized that both sleep duration and consistency are important factors for healthy aging outcomes. Their findings indicate that both increased *and* short sleep patterns are linked to a lower probability of successful aging.

As both excessive and insufficient sleep have been linked to adverse outcomes, most sleep experts recommend that adults sleep seven to nine hours a night, and that they maintain a regular sleep schedule. The REM stage of sleeping is when your body and brain processes and releases experiences and renews themselves, so the depth and quality of sleep is also important.

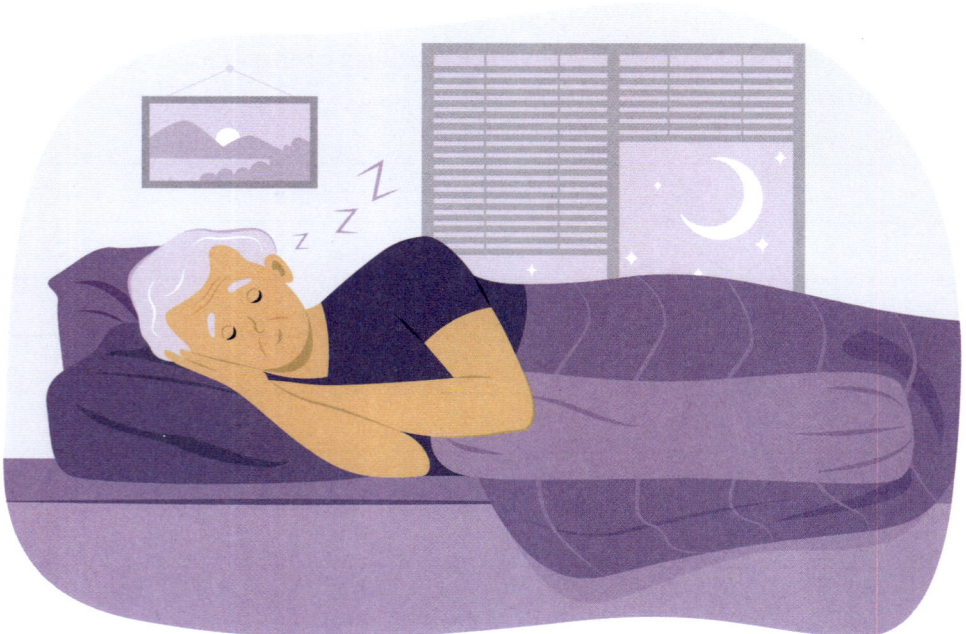

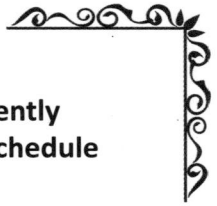

So, how well have you been sleeping lately? Do you consistently sleep seven to nine hours per night? Do you maintain this schedule on weekends? If not, how many hours are you sleeping?

_____

_____

_____

_____

_____

_____

_____

_____

_____

Do you fall asleep easily and wake up feeling refreshed, or are you waking often during the night and waking up most mornings feeling almost as tired as you were when you went to bed?

_____

_____

_____

_____

_____

_____

_____

_____

HEALTH BENEFITS OF SLEEP

While not getting enough sleep can cause serious medical issues, getting enough sleep helps you in a multitude of ways. When you sleep seven to nine hours on a regular schedule, it helps you:

- Get sick less often
- Stay at a healthy weight
- Reduce stress and improve your mood
- Improve your heart health and metabolism
- Lower your risk of chronic conditions such as;
    - Type 2 diabetes
    - Heart disease
    - High blood pressure
    - Stroke
- Lessen the risk of motor vehicle crashes and related injury or death
- Improve your attention and memory to better perform daily activities.

SO, HOW'S *YOUR* SLEEP QUALITY?

According to the National Sleep Foundation, all the dimensions of sleep quality can be self-rated following a night of your typical sleep pattern by using a checklist based on age. Answer 'yes' or 'no' to the following questions:

Adults (18-64 years old):

- Did you fall asleep in thirty minutes or less?
- Did you wake up one time or less during the night?
- In total, were you awake for twenty minutes or less after falling asleep?
- Were you mostly asleep while in bed (i.e., seven or eight hours)?

Older Adults (65 years or older):

- Did you fall asleep in thirty minutes or less?
- Did you wake two times or less during the night?
- In total, were you awake thirty minutes or less after falling asleep?
- Were you mostly asleep while in bed (i.e.,seven or eight hours)?

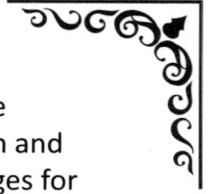

If you answered 'yes' to most of the questions, you likely have good sleep quality. If you answered mostly 'no,' focusing upon and improving how well you sleep will offer you the best advantages for good health going forward.

Seriously, do you sleep well most of the time? If not, what interferes?

_____

_____

_____

_____

What do you do to foster sound sleep?

_____

_____

_____

_____

_____

How many hours do you typically sleep at night? Does it feel sufficient? If not, what can you do to add time?

_____

_____

_____

_____

_____

IMPROVE YOUR SLEEP HABITS

Even if you scored pretty well on the current sleep patterns quiz, there are definite steps you can take to improve your sleep quality and establish the kind of habits that will serve you well and help you age gracefully. Consider them ways to fine-tune your sleep routine. If you practice them over time, you'll soon experience the positive health effects that getting a solid night's sleep provide.

Adhere to a Sleep Schedule. A regular schedule (yes, even on weekends) helps to sync your circadian rhythm, which dictates when you feel sleepy or awake and aids you in falling asleep faster and sleeping deeper. Aim to get seven to nine hours of sleep per night.

Prepare for Sleep. A bedtime routine carried out each night teaches your body that it's time to go to sleep. Consistent dinner times can also be an important cue for your circadian rhythm. Eating a light dinner two to three hours before bedtime gives your body time to fully digest the meal. Avoid heavy meals, and alcohol, both of which can disrupt sleep.

Transition into sleep mode. Try transitional activities—take a warm bath or shower, meditate, gently stretch, or read something soothing—to let your body know that it's time to fall asleep. Even smells can help, especially scents like lavender.

Turn out the lights. Dimming light prior to bed helps trigger your body's natural circadian rhythm. While sleeping, blackout curtains and blinds eliminate light pollution and remove outside light, creating a dark environment that's primed for sleep. If you have the ability, program your drapes to open, or a soft light to turn on, around daybreak. This helps your body awaken naturally.

Turn off electronics. Blue light prevents the natural production of melatonin, the chemical that tells your brain that it's time to sleep. Ideally, keep your bedroom free from televisions, tablets, phones, and laptops. At the very least, stop using them for at least an hour before you go to bed. If you like to read before bed, switching out your tablet or phone for a real book can help you fall asleep faster.

Create a sleep environment. A dark, cool bedroom that is free of distractions is the ideal place to get a good night of sleep. Find a comfortable mattress that supports your spine, and a pillow that best supports your neck. Invest in cozy bedding. If you're sensitive to temperature, find bedding designed to help you to maintain your ideal temperature. Keep the room between 60 to 67 degrees.

Use white noise. A white noise machine or even a small fan can mask unexpected sounds that might keep you, or startle you, awake.

Which of the above do you feel would be most effective for improving your sleep quality?

_____

_____

_____

_____

_____

_____

Which ones will you try?

_____

_____

_____

_____

_____

_____

YOU MAY NEED HELP IF . . .

If you have sleep apnea or any other ongoing sleep disturbance, it's best to discuss more specific strategies with your doctor. Common signs of sleep disorders include:

- Trouble falling or staying asleep, even after making healthy changes to your sleep routine

- Still feeling tired after sleeping the recommended number of hours

- Sleepiness that impedes everyday activities, like driving or concentrating at work

- Frequent loud snoring

- Pauses in breathing, or gasping while you sleep

- Tingling or crawling feelings in your legs or arms at night that feel better when you move or massage the area

- Feeling like it's hard to move when you first wake up.

If you have any of these signs, talk to a doctor or nurse. You may need testing or treatment for a sleep disorder.

WAKE UP TO SUNSHINE

Sunlight aids in the correct production of the stress hormone cortisol, which sets up your natural body clock for the day. Studies have found that getting just five to thirty minutes of direct morning sunlight on your face, two to three times a week, helps your body produce the adequate amount of Vitamin D3, which is crucial to health and energy. Exposure to sunlight within the first hour of waking up is found to improve focus, productivity, and energy. This is because sunlight encourages cortisol levels to be released at the appropriate time, which brings an extra boost of energy at the start of the day.

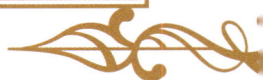

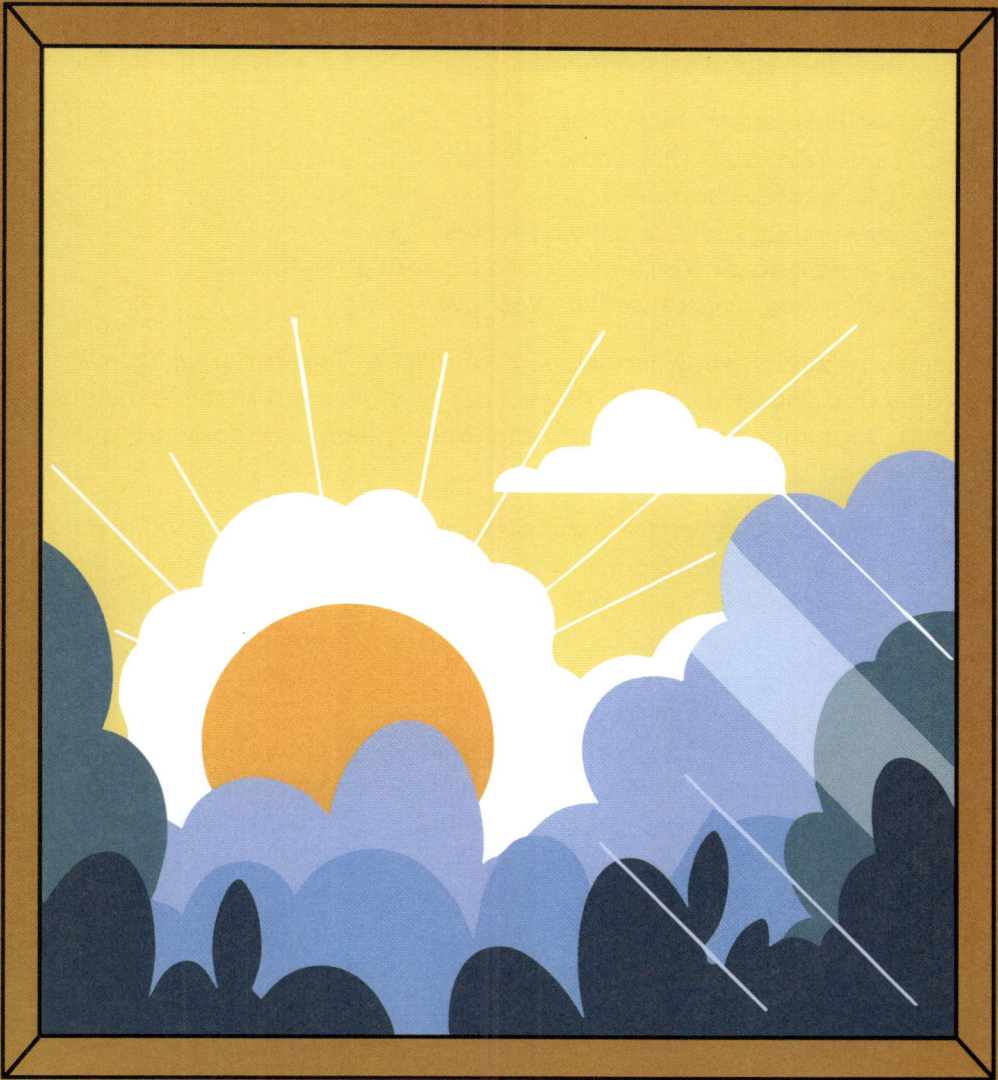

PRACTICE ESSENTIAL EXERCISE

As you age, the way you move can greatly affect your overall health and stamina. I suspect you've heard or read somewhere that 'sitting is the new smoking.' Scientists have found that those who fall into a sedentary lifestyle will age faster than those who move their body frequently. To maintain a strong, healthy body, it's essential to:

- Avoid sedentary behaviors
- Exercise at least three days a week
- Take a brisk walk daily
- Stay limber: practice daily stretches
- Use weights or resistance bands to strengthen muscles
- Find a new physical activity you love.

To keep your body strong, limber, and youthful well into your eighties, it's essential that you focus on the three types of movement that will maintain strength, endurance, and flexibility and thereby help your body more gracefully adjust to aging:

1. **Range of Motion or Flexibility:** Employ slow execution while putting all your joints through a full range of motion, plus flexion (bending) and extension. Taking yoga, Tai Chi, or Pilates classes would help you sustain flexibility, but slow, steady stretches you can do at home are fine.

2. **Toning and Muscle Building:** Regularly include weight-bearing exercises to help maintain and build muscle strength. Options for weight-bearing exercises are listed on page 100 but always check with a professional to make sure what you are doing is aligned to both benefit and protect your body type and skill level. Regular workouts are far more important than how much weight you lift or how hard you work out.

3. **Aerobic or Cardiorespiratory Work:** Make sure you get your heart rate up while exercising. It not only strengthens your heart and lungs, but gets blood flowing throughout your body and thereby also provides more energy and sharpens your mind. Running will likely be too stressful on your knees, but other weight-bearing activities are more than adequate for maintaining health. The list on page 100 is a good place to start.

It's more effective if you alternate the days when you do weight-bearing *activities* with the days you focus on weight-bearing *exercises*, and if you always remember to give your muscles time to rest between strenuous activities.

PUT IN THE TIME

As you age, aerobic exercise is fundamental for maintaining heart health, enhancing stamina, and managing a healthy weight. Activities that elevate the heart rate, even at a moderate intensity, contribute significantly to overall well-being and can reduce the risk of chronic diseases such as heart disease, obesity, and type 2 diabetes. Recommended guidelines suggest at least 150 minutes of moderate-intensity aerobic activity or 75 minutes of vigorous-intensity activity per week.

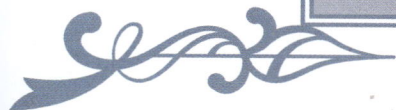

CHOOSE WEIGHT-BEARING ACTIVITIES

When you engage in weight-bearing activities, your body's weight bolsters the effect you get from the movement. Weight-bearing activities are essential to keeping your body strong, flexible, and functioning at peak capacity, particularly when you do them three days a week. There is a wide range of weight-bearing activities to choose from, such as:

- Brisk walking
- Climbing stairs
- Dancing
- Hiking
- Jogging
- Jumping rope
- Step aerobics
- Tennis or other racquet sports
- Pickleball
- House or yard work.

Before you leap into something particularly challenging, or if you have physical limitations, please ask your doctor which activities will most benefit your health and what the upper limits of each activity should be.

You'll also want to specifically add *weight-bearing exercises*, which have been shown to greatly benefit your body—and your brain. Some you may want to do in a health club with supervision, but you can also do many at home, including:

- Elastic resistance bands
- Free weights
- Weight machines
- Push-ups or planks
- Squats
- Balance exercises.

Which of the preceding activities or exercises most appeal to you?

_____

_____

_____

_____

_____

_____

_____

Which will you commit to adopting as a habit?

_____

_____

_____

_____

_____

_____

_____

Caution: Always discuss any new activity with your health professional. And if you have specific challenges or any concerns, consult a physical therapist who can offer suggestions and help design a program that will provide steady progress, without injury.

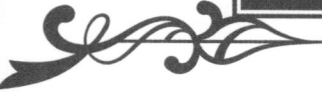

FIND YOUR EXERCISE BUDDIES

At the *New York Times* Well Festival in 2025, Kelly McGonigal, a health psychologist at Stanford University and the author of the book *The Joy of Movement*, said one reason exercising with friends makes us happy is that it helps foster connection to others. Even if the idea makes you self-conscious, try joining a running club or attending a Zumba class, "When we move in sync with other people, our bodies enter a state—our brains enter a state that neuroscientists call 'we mode,'" Dr. McGonigal said. "We enter a state of togetherness that is biologically real, and we can sense it as a kind of trust and closeness and belonging."

PROTECT YOUR SKIN

Too much exposure to the sun's ultraviolet (UV) rays is a major risk factor for most skin cancers. If your unprotected skin sunburns after an hour in the sun, you are considered sun sensitive and need to use some form of sun protection every day. Obviously, avoiding long exposure during the hottest hours of the day, between 10 a.m. and 4 p.m., and using sunscreen on any exposed skin is paramount, but you can also:

- Primarily stay in the shade

- Wear a wide-brimmed hat

- Wear clothing to the ankles

- Wear a long-sleeved shirt.

If avoiding skin cancer isn't sufficient motivation to protect your skin, UV sun exposure is directly to blame for about 80 percent of the visible signs of wrinkles and aging skin.

YOUR COMMITMENTS TO PHYSICAL HEALTH

Use the space below to record your commitments to improving your physical health in the interest of an easier path to aging. Be specific about what you want to do and what you will immediately commit to incorporating into your lifestyle.

PROTECT YOUR BRAIN

Your brain function has everything to do with aging gracefully. If you want to keep neurons growing and firing, your cortexes alert and focused, and both your short- and long-term memory viable, you need to adopt and sustain habits that protect and nurture your brain *now*. Eating well nourishes your brain, exercising on a regular basis keeps essential blood and oxygen flowing, and sleeping well gives your brain sufficient time to cleanse and refresh. All are *essential* if you want to maintain peak functioning—and you do—but there are other things you can do to nourish and protect your brain.

Your brain is composed of billions of neurons: nerve cells that collect, process, and transmit information, as well as a complex network of electrical circuits that allow these neurons to 'talk' with one another. These connections are crucial, as neurons in the brain also can send messages to other parts of the body through the nervous system. Neuroplasticity is your brain's ability to form and reconfigure this vast network of neural connections. When we're young, our brains are still growing, producing new neurons at a rapid pace. By the time we enter our late twenties, our brains have begun steadily, if slowly, losing brain cells. The rate of shrinkage increases after sixty, which begins to affect cognitive functions like memory, processing speed, decision-making and learning, all the areas that may leave you feeling a little less sharp as you get older.

Though the number of neurons may decline with age, emerging research has shown that neuroplasticity helps the brain retain its ability to adapt both structurally and functionally *throughout life.* In short, neuroplasticity means that your brain can still produce new neurons, and that you can retrain your brain, tap into new skills, and maybe even learn a new language, no matter your age.

Research suggests that the phrase 'use it or lose it' applies to your brain and cognitive abilities. To use neuroplasticity to your advantage, especially as you age, it's important to regularly stimulate your brain. The more stimulating habits you cultivate, the better. Research suggests that the benefits of these activities accrue over your lifetime.

In a study reported by *The Journal of Neuropsychiatry and Clinical Neurosciences*, Mayo Clinic researchers identified the top five activities shown to help maintain brain function:

1. Regular social engagement, featuring in-depth conversations
2. Craft activities (knitting, quilting, woodwork, painting, gardening etc.)
3. Playing games, particularly novel ones, in social settings
4. Reading books, particularly challenging ones
5. Computer activities, particularly stimulating ones.

Social activities, such as traveling, were marginally significant. Even though the point-estimates for reading magazines, playing music, artistic activities, and group activities were associated with reduced odds of having mild cognitive impairment (MCI), none of these reached statistical significance. The equally high prevalence of reading newspapers in both groups yielded no significant between-group difference. [*The Journal of Neuropsychiatry and Clinical Neurosciences*, Volume 23, Number 2; https://doi.org/10.1176/jnp.23.2.jnp149]

Though your brain regularly needs greater stimulation than they provide, traditional brain-training activities such as puzzles (crossword, Sudoku, jigsaw) and other games that rely on logic, math, language, and visuospatial skills can help to challenge various cognitive abilities, improving processing speed and mental agility. Look online for games *specifically designed* to boost cognitive skills. At age fifty, you can join AARP and find many brain-stimulating games available on their website. Just be sure that you're also incorporating the activities mentioned in the list above, particularly anything that is both novel and challenging.

Do you participate in any of the above activities? If not, what do you do?

_____

_____

_____

_____

List any activities that you would enjoy that would help you strengthen neuronal connections and help your brain maintain peak functioning.

Which new activities are you willing to explore?

_____

_____

_____

_____

_____

_____

_____

_____

_____

_____

_____

_____

ANOTHER POTENT REASON TO EXERCISE

Regular physical activity has been shown to contribute to the primary, secondary, and tertiary prevention of cognitive decline and dementia. A study of 128,925 adults determined that rates of cognitive decline were twice as common in sedentary people who didn't exercise much, if at all.

(Alzheimer's Association, 2018; 2018 Physical Activity Guidelines Advisory Committee, 2018; Baumgart et al., 2015)

STIMULATE YOUR BRAIN

The best way to stimulate your brain varies from one person to another. If you choose activities that take you slightly outside of your comfort zone, you're giving your brain a workout. Consider the following brain-stimulating possibilities.

- Play cards or board games, especially if they're complicated *and* unfamiliar to you.

- Take lifelong learning classes to explore a challenging, new-to-you topic.

- Go to lectures on a multitude of topics.

- Read books that challenge you to think.

- Learn a new language, musical instrument, or skill.

- Knit, quilt, sew, or construct objects using complicated patterns.

- Take up a new, challenging art or craft.

- Plan a detailed trip itinerary to a new vacation spot.

- Try new, complicated recipes on a regular basis.

- Host regular dinner parties that encourage deep discussions.

- Host your own monthly book, hobby, or game club.

"On the whole, age comes more gently to those who have some doorway into an abstract world—art, or philosophy, or learning—regions where the years are scarcely noticed and the young and old can meet in a pale truthful light."

— FREYA STARK, EXPLORER

Take note that the word 'new' appears in most of the mentioned examples. That's key because *novel experiences* help stimulate the growth of new brain connections. Ideally, challenge your brain in many ways and continually change your methods up.

After viewing the list, which activities most appeal? Pick three that you'll commit to trying.

1

_____

_____

_____

2

_____

_____

_____

3

_____

_____

_____

Can you think of any other activities that you'd like to add?

_____

_____

_____

_____

_____

_____

PERK UP!

One of the most accessible and easiest ways to perk up your brain is to practice mindfulness. Mindfulness is not merely a coping mechanism that will help you navigate the physiological and psychological stressors of aging; it is an active intervention that directly enhances cognitive function, including memory and brain connections. Mindfulness meditation can lead to decreases in markers of cellular aging, reduced distress, and improved mood and thinking skills. Regularly practicing mindfulness can actively re-wire your brain, improve emotional resilience, and reduce modifiable midlife risk factors for Alzheimer's disease, such as high blood pressure and cholesterol. Think of it as an essential tool for perking up your brain and building cognitive resilience, that also contributes to overall well-being and longevity.

When you meditate, you are essentially practicing the art of mindfulness, a technique that trains your brain to focus solely on what is happening in the present moment by increasing awareness of feelings, thoughts, or bodily sensations. In mindfulness meditation, rather than focusing on thoughts, the goal is to focus on your breath, take note of thoughts that arise, but quickly release them, and resume focus on your breathing. After you've completed your meditation, it may be helpful to recall any patterns in thought and figure out why they are constantly interrupting or distracting you. The process of mindfully dismissing thoughts during meditation can help your brain learn to better resist getting caught up in ruminative or other negative thought patterns. Mindfulness also helps you recognize thoughts you need to consciously jettison, such as unrealistic fears.

Nonjudgmentally and compassionately focusing solely on what you're seeing, hearing, smelling, thinking, feeling, witnessing, or experiencing in the *present* moment, while choosing to dismiss distracting thoughts, keeps your brain more agile and helps tamp down stress. If practiced often enough, over time, mindfulness becomes ingrained.

HOW TO MINDFULLY MEDITATE

All you need to practice mindfulness is five minutes and a quiet spot where you can sit at least relatively undisturbed in a meditative state. To start, simply move into a sitting position (on the floor or on a chair with your feet on the floor to ground yourself is fine) and begin by focusing all your attention on a single focal point (a lit candle, for example), or simply close your eyes and focus your attention on your breath, noticing how it feels moving through your body as you slowly inhale and exhale. As thoughts arise (and many will!), immediately release them (view them as butterflies flitting in and out of consciousness), and resume focusing on your focal point or breathing.

Work your way up to fifteen to twenty minutes of daily meditation. It's helpful to use a timer, and to make mindfulness meditation a habit. The more you practice, the sooner it will be a "muscle memory" you can automatically use when you feel stressed. Because mindfulness meditation will help you learn to pay closer attention to what's happening to you and around you, in the present moment, it will help you keep your brain more alert.

The following mindfulness meditations will get you started. Once you've done these, you can find a multitude of guided mindfulness meditations online or come up with your own ideas. Remember, you don't have to officially be sitting cross-legged on a cushion in a meditative state. Mindfulness is simply paying attention to what's happening in the present, and it can be done when sitting anywhere, walking, cooking, dancing, or lying in bed. All you have to do is focus solely on the sensory experiences that occur while you are doing whatever you are doing, allowing all your senses to awaken and dismissing intrusive thoughts that detract from the present moment.

THE THREE-MINUTE MINDFULNESS MEDITATION

Find a quiet place to sit down and close your eyes. Slowly breathe in and out until you feel calm.

First: Spend a minute noticing what's happening inside. When thoughts arise, immediately release them. What emotions or feelings are you experiencing? Don't judge them, just notice them and how they feel in your body. Notice sensations in your body and identify them as pleasure, joy, tension, pain, discomfort, alertness, and so on.

Second: Spend the next minute focusing solely on your breathing. Notice how deeply and slowly inhaling and exhaling affects your lungs and the rise and fall of your abdomen. If thoughts intrude, send them flitting away and return focus to your breathing.

Third: Spend the last minute expanding your attention. Notice how slow, deep breathing is affecting your whole body. Notice how nourishing breath feels, how the steady rhythm relaxes body and brain. If you notice any areas of tension or pain, focus on the area and breathe into and around it. If your focus wanes, bring it back to your body and any new sensations.

After three minutes, slowly open your eyes and take a cleansing breath.

How did you do as far as dismissing thoughts and keeping your attention focused, first on your breathing, and later feelings or bodily sensations?

What was the nature of thoughts that occurred? Is there a discernable pattern of thoughts? If so, are these typical of how your brain gets caught up in a thought loop?

Were you able to keep redirecting your attention back to solely what you were experiencing in the mediative moment?

THE LOVING KINDNESS MEDITATION

This is a great meditation to help calm yourself and generate loving feelings. Simply sit still, close your eyes, breathe slowly in and out, and then bring your awareness to your heart and imagine that you can breathe energy into your heart. Now, bring yourself into mind with warmth and kindness, then make four loving wishes:

May I be safe   May I be happy   May I be well   May I live with ease

Pause between each wish to take note of any feelings or thoughts that arise, but don't allow them to distract you. Maintain focus on offering loving kindness to yourself. If you need to write the wishes down, it's okay to have a list you refer to during meditation, at least until it becomes ingrained. If you make up your own wishes, that's fine, too.

Repeat the same meditation for a loved one or friend, simply by bringing that person to mind and then repeating each wish for them. Pause between each wish to take note of any feelings or thoughts that arise, but don't focus on them. Keep your focus on offering loving kindness.

To close, repeat the same meditation for someone you have encountered but don't know personally (the barista at Starbucks, a librarian, or a fellow church member, for example). Pause between each wish to take note of any feelings or thoughts that arise, but don't focus on them. Keep your focus on offering loving kindness.

Close by bringing your attention back to your breath. If any thoughts or feelings arise take note of what they are so you can write about them upon completion.

How did this meditation feel? Were you able to feel and extend loving kindness? If not, what blocked your efforts?

_____

If you experienced loving feelings, how did they feel in your body?

_____

HAPPY MEMORY MEDITATION

Once you are settled, focus on your breathing and bring up a memory of an event that brought you great happiness. Try to see the memory as a movie taking place in your mind. Focus on re-experiencing the feelings, sounds, tastes, smells, colors, or whatever senses bolster the memory. Allow yourself to feel as if it's all happening again. Stick with this process for ten minutes, bringing your focus back if it wanders.

How did it feel to recall such a happy memory? What brought it fully to life for you? What about this *particular* memory made it such a happy one?

_____

_____

_____

_____

_____

_____

_____

_____

_____

_____

_____

_____

_____

_____

_____

_____

_____

_____

Make a list of happy events in your life that you could call up when needed. Jot down details that will evoke the memory.

Note: The next time you feel anxious, it's helpful to use this mediation to calm your mind.

You can mindfully mediate anywhere. If you're taking a walk outside, for example, look up into the trees and notice small details: Are the leaves wet from recent rain, spring green or changing colors, drying out from a lack of rain? How are they shaped? Is the tree bark dark or light, smooth or thick and scaly? Can you see birds in the branches? How does the sunlight look filtering through the leaves? How does it sound when a breeze sends the leaves fluttering? Can you hear or smell anything? Are there insects or birds making noise? How is your body feeling during this experience?

Mindfulness trains your brain to consciously pay nonjudgmental attention to a point of focus, making sure that anytime your mind wanders, you bring it back to the original focus. Different ways of meditating include the use of mantras, positive self-talk, and controlled breathing exercises.

TRY CONTROLLED BREATHING

To control your breathing, breathe from your diaphragm, not your chest. Pull the air in through your nose all the way down into your belly, then exhale with your stomach first, using your diaphragm to push the air out of your lungs. Only your stomach should move, not your chest. The inhale should be a long, continuous breath (at least to the count of eight), followed by a pause before exhaling (at least to the count of eight), and then another eight-second pause before the next inhale. This slow, steady breathing can help control your heart rate and allow your mind to relax. It's also an effective way to reduce anxiety.

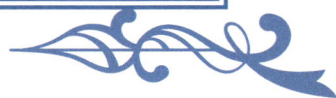

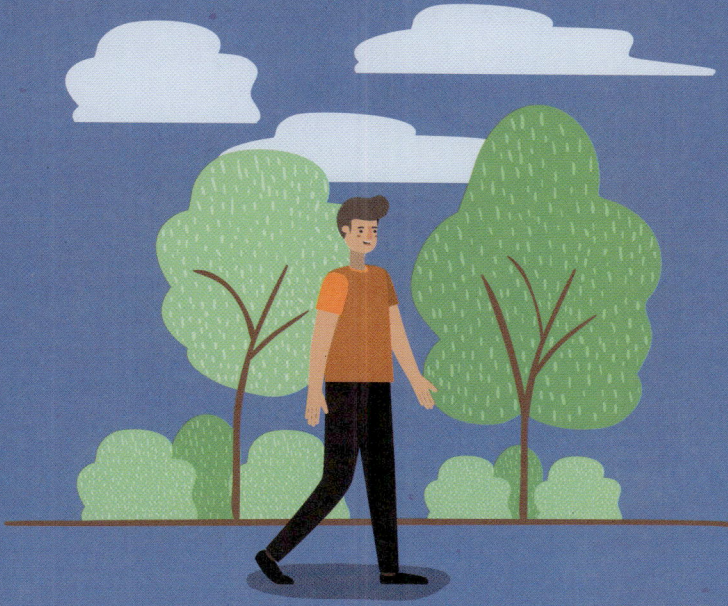

"Mindfulness practice means that we commit fully in each moment to be present; inviting ourselves to interface with this moment in full awareness, with the intention to embody as best we can an orientation of calmness, mindfulness, and equanimity right here and right now."

— JON KABAT-ZINN, *WHEREVER YOU GO, THERE YOU ARE: MINDFULNESS MEDITATION IN EVERYDAY LIFE*

WHY SOCIAL INTERACTION MATTERS

In an article in *Healthy Aging*, Amit A. Shah, MD, a geriatrician, internist, and palliative care specialist at the Mayo Clinic, stressed the importance of having and maintaining strong social connections for the health of your brain. "Interacting with others is exercise for your brain—it's one of the best ways to improve your cognitive flexibility. It's likely more beneficial than doing crossword puzzles or other brain games."

The reason it's so essential to brain health is that interacting socially keeps a multitude of neurons firing and connecting, helping you learn new things and form new memories, all of which stimulate many different areas of cognition, such as executive function, thought generation, spatial function, and memory. Essentially, interacting with others provides a workout for your brain.

"I tell my patients: 'Action is important,'" says Dr. Shah. "It can be hard, and sometimes intimidating, to be in social situations, but you have to do it. It takes effort to learn about a new person or make a new connection, but it's very important to cognition," he continues. "Think of it as a workout for your soul, your happiness, and your brain health."

We'll discuss social engagement in depth later but pause a moment to assess how well you are doing socially. Do you have five or more friends? Do you see them often? When was the last time you expanded your social base? If you're not being social, why not? What's holding you back?

_____

_____

_____

_____

_____

_____

_____

_____

SING!

While simply listening to music or a story is a fabulous way to relax, it can ramp down your energy. Some evidence suggests, however, that making music helps boost energy levels. A study published in 2018 found that people who actively made music through singing, keyboard playing, or rhythm tapping felt more energetic than others. Singing also gives you a kind of emotional high and reduces levels of stress hormones in your body. The next time you listen to a song, try singing along to feel energized.

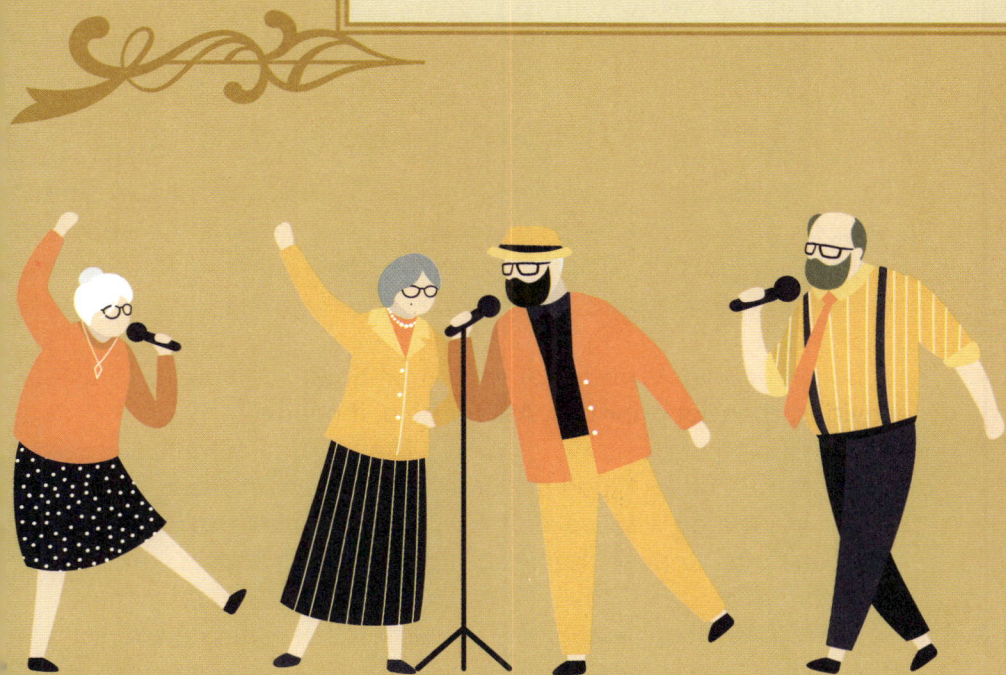

BOOST YOUR ENERGY

Your body is more than just the vehicle for your brain. Once you start inhabiting it, paying attention to it, nurturing it, and moving it, you'll soon recognize how powerful your body can be, and how much capacity you can generate to energetically move through life.

Exercise is a natural energy booster, because whenever you do it, oxygen-rich blood surges through your body to your heart, muscles, and brain. Even if you can spare only ten minutes, regularly squeezing a workout into your day will help keep your energy levels at their peak. Also, simply move around every chance you get, even if it's just pacing while you're on the phone. Exercise also positively impacts sleep which, in turn, boosts energy levels.

Exercise not only gives your cells more energy to burn, it boosts your mood, too. Exercise releases dopamine and endorphins that contribute to greater feelings of well-being and a 'natural high.' So, when you're feeling a little low on energy, don't skip that gym session, as you could be missing out on impressive mental and energy gains.

In addition to boosting your energy by getting sufficient sleep, staying physically active, and feeding your body well, the Harvard Medical School has also identified five *specific* actions you can take to boost energy.

1. **Control stress.** Stress saps energy. Talk with a friend or relative, join a support group, see a psychotherapist, or try meditation, self-hypnosis, yoga, and Tai Chi, all of which reduce stress. You can also practice mindfulness meditation. Whatever you choose, make defusing stress a daily habit.
2. **Lighten your load.** Whether at work or at home, streamline 'must-do' activities, then set priorities. Ask for help, if needed.
3. **Avoid smoking or excessive drinking.** The nicotine in tobacco speeds the heart rate, raises blood pressure, and stimulates brain-wave activity associated with wakefulness, making it harder to fall asleep. Marijuana often induces laziness, and alcohol is a depressant, not a stimulant.
4. **Eat for energy.** Foods with a low glycemic index maintain energy levels longer. These include whole grains, high-fiber vegetables, nuts, and healthy oils such as olive oil. Proteins and fats have glycemic

indexes that are as low as you can go, close to zero. Most carbohydrates and processed foods have a high glycemic index.
5. Drink water. One of the first signs of dehydration is fatigue. Water is the *sole nutrient* that has been shown to enhance performance for all but the most demanding endurance activities.

These are all behaviors that you will want to foster, as making them habits will help you feel and see yourself as an energetic person, even well into your nineties.

How's your average energy level? If it's regularly flagging, do you know why?

_____

_____

What changes could you make to bolster your energy? Which ones are you willing to make a habit?

_____

_____

FIRE UP YOUR ENERGY WITH AEROBICS

There's clear evidence that even moderate exercise can make you more energetic. University of Georgia researchers found that sedentary people who complained of fatigue were able to increase their energy levels by 20 percent and decrease their fatigue by 65 percent by engaging in regular, low-intensity exercise like aerobic workouts (see page 99). Study author Patrick J. O'Connor, a professor of kinesiology at University of Georgia, attributes the energy boost to "exercise-induced changes in activity in brain neurons and circuits that underlie feelings of energy and fatigue. It's likely that neurotransmitters like norepinephrine, dopamine and histamine are part of the process."

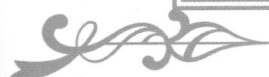

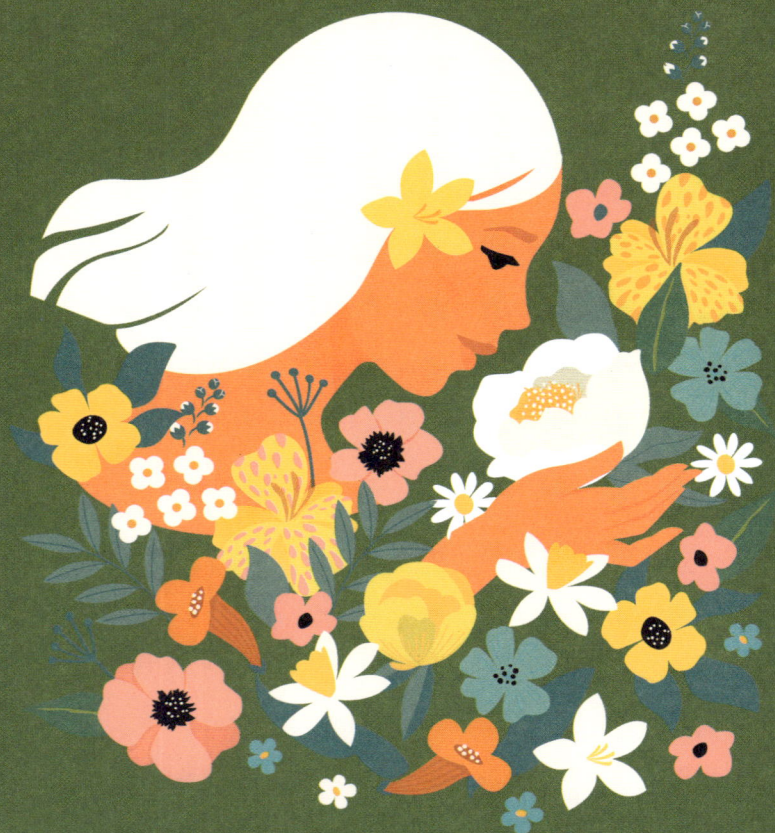

You don't stop laughing when you grow old,
you grow old when you stop laughing.

— GEORGE BERNARD SHAW

KEY TAKEAWAYS FOR *NOURISH YOUR BRAIN AND BODY*

- Aging brings inevitable changes to the body and brain, but how well you age depends greatly on the healthy habits you adopt and maintain, especially starting in midlife. By focusing on your remaining strengths and committing to essentials like nutritious food, good sleep, physical activity, mental engagement, and energy renewal, you can age with vitality and purpose.

- Genetics influence how we age, but lifestyle choices—especially diet—play a critical role in determining long-term health outcomes, with studies showing that those who eat mostly plant-based, minimally processed foods have a significantly higher chance of aging without chronic disease. Getting seven to nine hours of sleep each night on a regular schedule supports overall health by strengthening the immune system, managing weight, improving mood, and boosting heart and metabolic function.

- Staying physically active is essential to maintaining strength, flexibility, and endurance, all of which help slow the aging process and support overall health. Maintaining a healthy, adaptable brain is key to aging well, and habits like eating well, exercising, sleeping sufficiently, and regularly stimulating your mind can preserve cognitive function and support neuroplasticity (brain flexibility) throughout life. Engaging in mentally challenging and socially inter-active activities—such as crafting, reading, playing games, and deep conversations—helps keep neural pathways active and supports your brain's ability to learn, adapt, and grow, even as you age.

- Mindfulness is a powerful, accessible tool that enhances cognitive function, emotional resilience, and overall brain health by helping you stay present, reduce stress, and rewire negative thought patterns. Regular mindfulness meditation can slow markers of aging, lower midlife risk factors for Alzheimer's, and improve memory, mood, and mental clarity—making it a key practice for long-term well-being and cognitive longevity.

"When you are a young person, you are like a young creek, and you meet many rocks, many obstacles and difficulties on your way. You hurry to get past these obstacles and get to the ocean. But as the creek moves down through the fields, it becomes larger and calmer, and it can enjoy the reflection of the sky. It's wonderful. You will arrive at the sea anyway so enjoy the journey. Enjoy the sunshine, the sunset, the moon, the birds, the trees, and the many beauties along the way. Taste every moment of your daily life."

— THÍCH NHẤT HẠNH,
GOOD CITIZENS: CREATING ENLIGHTENED SOCIETY

FIND
Purpose
AND
Meaning

Find Purpose and Meaning

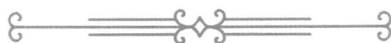

Surgeon, medical professor, and author on the meaning of life, Atul Gawande (*Being Mortal; The Checklist Manifesto*) argues that in Western societies, medicine has created the ideal conditions for transforming aging into an undesirable "long, slow fade." He believes channeling our resources towards biological survival has led to us overlooking the importance that quality of life plays.

Multiple studies reveal that having a purpose in later life contributes to a longer, happier life and that people who view the aging process as a potential for personal growth are more likely to be healthy in their seventies and eighties. In fact, those who think of themselves as 'still young,' retained more cognitive and physical abilities than those who 'feel old.'

Having a perceived purpose in life provides meaning. Beyond being a healthy, loving partner and parent, a reliable and valuable employee, or a good friend, having a purpose motivates you to focus on and strive to be the best you possible. When you identify and choose your purpose, living with purpose provides the meaning needed to fuel enthusiasm throughout life and thereby keeps you active and engaged. So how do you identify your purpose? Begin by identifying your values.

IDENTIFY YOUR VALUES

Finding meaning in life is often considered synonymous with finding happiness, but meaning will only lead to happiness if it creates a purpose sufficient to motivate you to achieve your goals. To find meaning, you have to examine how you've been living your life thus far and evaluate how successful you've been at incorporating and honoring purpose and meaning. Going forward, it's important to both identify and clarify the values that motivate you to be your best self, or that bring you true fulfillment.

Living with purpose and meaning requires that you do more than profess your values. You need to be clear about what you believe and hold important, and then make sure your intentions, words, thoughts, and behaviors align with those beliefs. To achieve purpose and meaning, your actions need to be congruous with your values.

Here's a comprehensive list of core values to help you identify the ones that hold the most meaning for you, both now and going forward:

Authenticity	Fame	Peace
Achievement	Friendships	Pleasure
Adventure	Fun	Popularity
Authority	Growth	Recognition
Autonomy	Happiness	Religion
Balance	Honesty	Reputation
Beauty	Humor	Respect
Boldness	Influence	Responsibility
Compassion	Inner Harmony	Security
Challenge	Justice	Self-Respect
Citizenship	Kindness	Service
Community	Knowledge	Spirituality
Competency	Leadership	Stability
Contribution	Learning	Success
Creativity	Love	Status
Curiosity	Loyalty	Trustworthiness
Determination	Meaningful Work	Wealth
Fairness	Openness	Wisdom
Faith	Optimism	

Take time to deeply ponder each item above and then highlight the values that mean the most to you. If you like, highlight your present values in yellow, and those you most want to honor going forward in green (or another color). You can also use checkmarks or asterisks.

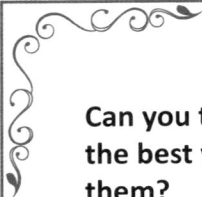

Can you think of any values not on the list that motivate you to be the best you possible? What are they and how do you manifest them?

_____

_____

_____

_____

_____

_____

_____

Have your values changed throughout your life? If so, how? Is your current lifestyle in alignment with your values?

_____

_____

_____

_____

_____

_____

_____

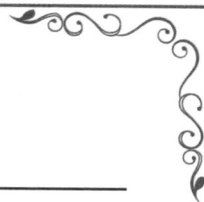

How does it feel to be you at this moment in time?

_____

_____

_____

_____

_____

Are you mostly happy and fulfilled, or often frustrated and unhappy or stressed? Why?

_____

_____

_____

_____

_____

What in your life brings you the greatest pleasure?

_____

_____

_____

_____

_____

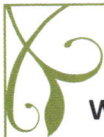

What in your life is most meaningful to you?

_____

_____

_____

_____

_____

What would you rather be doing?

_____

_____

_____

_____

_____

If you could do anything, pursue any path, what would it be?

_____

_____

_____

_____

_____

How could you make that happen?

_____

_____

_____

_____

_____

_____

_____

_____

_____

_____

_____

_____

GIVE ME THAT OLD TIME RELIGION

A 2018 study reported in Newsweek _found that people who have a strong religious or spiritual belief system lived four years longer than average. Note that longevity was not connected to any religion, only to a strong, faith-based belief._

YOUR QUEST FOR MEANING AND PURPOSE

To live a meaningful life, you need a plan. Your goals require plans, too. Understanding yourself as a whole person can lead to accomplishing big goals. With greater self-awareness, you can establish your strengths and use them to the best advantage.

To find meaning and purpose in your life, incorporate the following approaches:

1. Accept happiness as something *you* can create

2. Figure out what's missing in your life and find a way to incorporate it

3. Shake up your routine and try new activities

4. Commit to something you've always wanted to do

5. Connect with people with whom you share interests

6. Find new ways to use your natural talents

7. Set goals that are clear and challenging but achievable

8. Follow your internal compass when making decisions

9. Seek inspiration in books, lectures, or podcasts

10. Protect your physical well-being and mental health by pacing yourself

11. Make helping others something you love to do.

Highlight the suggestions above that you will commit to incorporating into your daily life (or list anything you can think of that's not in the above suggestions), then write about how you will take action that reinforces purpose and meaning.

_____

_____

_____

_____

_____

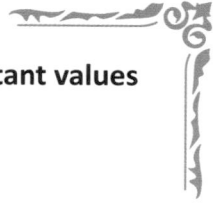

List at least five ways you can incorporate your most important values into your current life.

1
_____

2
_____

3
_____

4
_____

5
_____

GET FIRED UP

Try setting a goal to learn something new. Make the goal achievable and then put it into motion. Keep applying yourself until you reach the goal. Repeatedly doing this creates the ability to identify and maximize a motivational purpose. Without a motivational purpose that drives you forward to completion, it's easier to abandon goals and set plans aside.

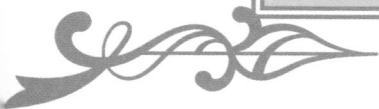

- When modern medicine prioritizes mere survival over quality of life, it may create a prolonged decline in aging, but it does not necessarily foster opportunities to fully live a meaningful later life. Research shows that having a sense of purpose and viewing aging as an opportunity for growth leads to improved health, sustained cognitive function, and increased happiness—especially when that purpose is grounded in clearly identified personal values and lived through aligned actions.

- Living a meaningful life starts with self-awareness of your values and deepest desires, as well as intentional planning to fulfill them. Anything that helps you leverage your strengths and set purposeful, achievable goals will provide the drive needed to live an active, fulfilling, healthier, and happier life.

- By identifying what brings you joy, shaking up your routine, connecting with others, and aligning your actions with your values, you can create a life filled with purpose, fulfillment, and lasting motivation, all of which will help you age gracefully.

"You will come to know things that can only be known with the wisdom of age and the grace of years. Most of those things will have to do with forgiveness."

— CHERYL STRAYED,
TINY BEAUTIFUL THINGS: ADVICE ON LOVE AND LIFE FROM DEAR SUGAR

"Our individual relationships are an untapped resource—a source of healing hiding in plain sight. They can help us live healthier, more productive, and more fulfilled lives. Answer that phone call from a friend. Make time to share a meal. Listen without the distraction of your phone. Perform an act of service. Express yourself authentically. The keys to human connection are simple, but extraordinarily powerful."

— FORMER UNITED STATES SURGEON GENERAL VIVEK MURTHY

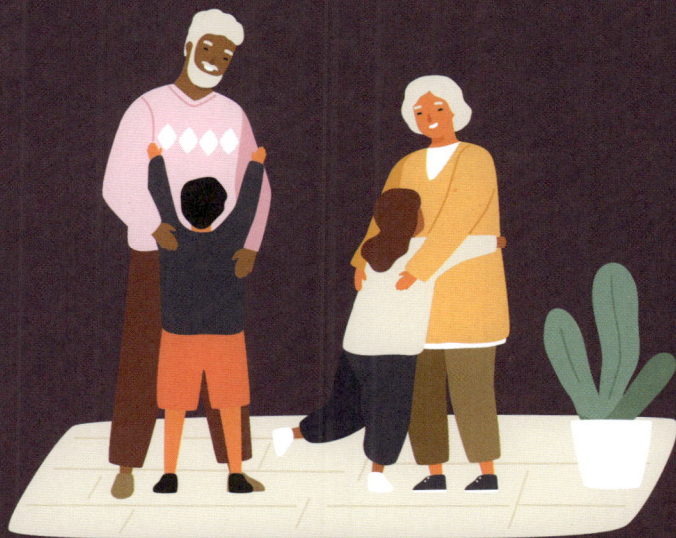

"Now that I'm older I know who I want to spend time with and who I don't. And that is one of the great things about getting older — it just clears out so much space. I want to be with my mom, my kids, and the people who fill my tank. And everybody else, I wish them well."

— REESE WITHERSPOON

EXPAND YOUR WORLD:
Cultivate Relationships

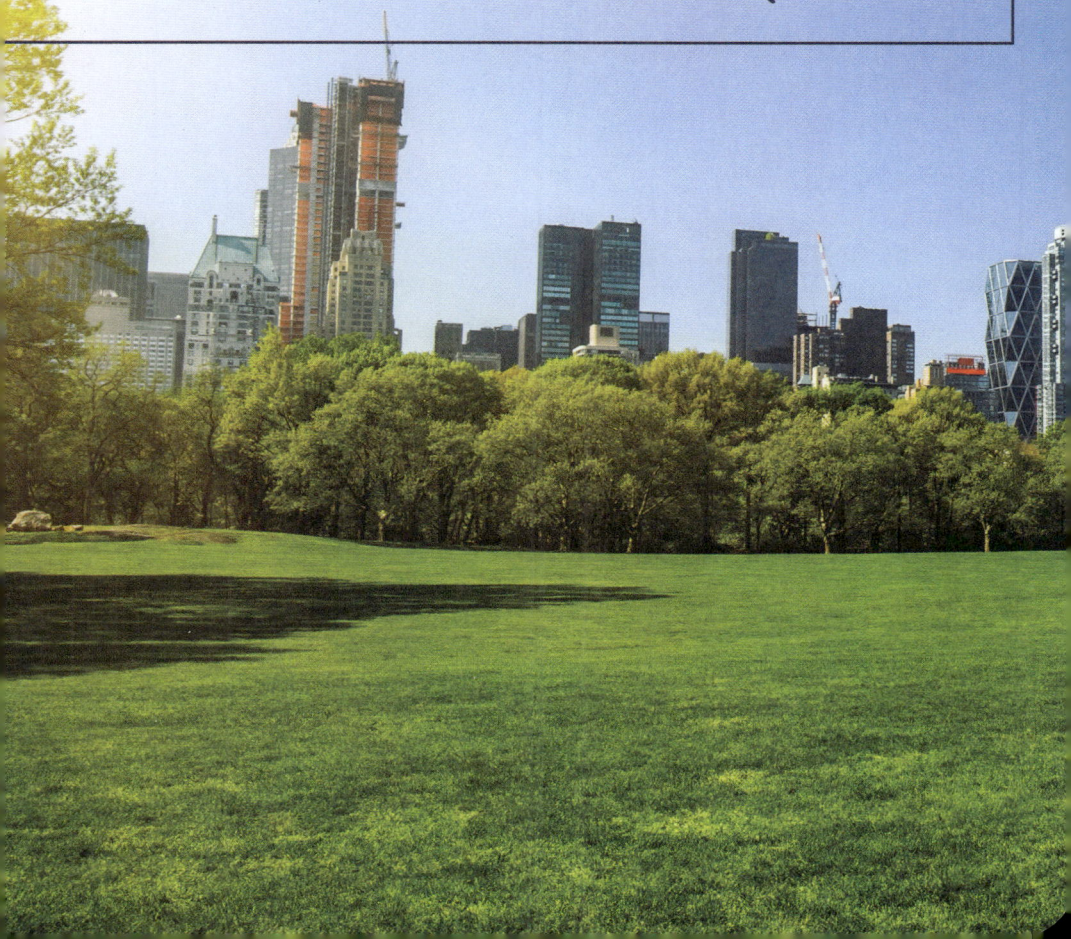

Expand Your World:
Cultivate Relationships

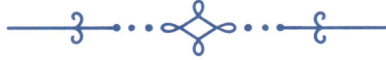

According to Mayo Clinic studies, in addition to essential support, establishing and maintaining *positive* relationships is good for your health. Relationships can boost your happiness, reduce stress, improve confidence and help you cope with traumatic events. Adults with a strong social network have a reduced risk of depression, lower blood pressure, and tend to maintain a healthier body mass index (BMI). Having a strong social network is essential to combating the increasing problem of loneliness and isolation, which are significant risk factors for depression, anxiety, cognitive decline, and even reduced longevity.

In an article in *Healthy Aging*, Amit A. Shah, MD, a geriatrician, internist and palliative care specialist at Mayo Clinic, emphasized the importance of social connections. "Over many years of taking care of older patients, I've learned that the factors many people think are most important for aging well—such as having longevity in your family or lack of physical illnesses—do not guarantee a positive experience with getting older, It's the quality, duration and nature of your relationships that seem to matter most."

Forming and maintaining a strong social network contributes to your ability to enjoy a longer, healthier life. A social network—made up of friends, family, co-workers, neighbors and others—provides opportunities for you to give and receive both instrumental and emotional support.

- Instrumental support is the tangible help you give or receive through physical acts of kindness, such as providing transportation for a neighbor to an appointment or offering childcare for friends or family.
- Emotional support is listening or closely observing needs and taking actions intended to lift someone's spirits, relieve sadness, give encouragement or offer advice.

How many close friends do you currently have and how long have they been close friends? Do you interact often with them, and do these interactions involve extensive conversation and/or joint activities? If you don't have close friends, why not?

_____

_____

Do you share intimate details of your life with all your friends? If not, who is your confidante (aside from your partner or spouse)? When having a difficult conversation with them, do you feel fully seen, heard, and supported? If not, why not? What's missing?

_____

_____

Do you regularly get together with your friends for social occasions? Do you offer them your full attention? Does interacting with them provide the kind of healthy back-and-forth conversations and actions that increase intimacy? If so, what fosters intimacy? If not, why?

_____

_____

When is the last time you made a new friend outside of work? Who and how did that happen? What could you do to make more friends?

_____

_____

Has something changed in your life that makes it hard to make friends or get together with friends? What is it and how can you address it?

_____

_____

THE THREE ASPECTS OF SOCIAL CONNECTION

Social connection can encompass the interactions, relationships, roles, and sense of connection individuals, communities, or society may experience. Your level of social connection is not determined simply by the number of close relationships you have, but in these three ways:

1. **Structural**: The number of relationships, variety of relationships (co-workers, friends, family, neighbors), and frequency of interactions you have with others. Household size, friend circle size, and marital/partner status affect your structural connection.

How would you rate your life in terms of structural relationships? Do you have enough variety? Where do you need to find more friends? Where or how could you make that happen?

_____

_____

2. **Functional**: The degree to which you can rely on others for various needs, such as emotional support, mentorship, or help in a crisis.

Do you have enough functional relationships? Who provides emotional support on a regular basis? List five people to whom you feel close enough to call upon when you need help or support. If you don't call on intimate friends when needed, why?

_____

_____

3. **Qualitative**: The degree to which relationships and interactions with others are positive, helpful, or satisfying, versus negative, unhelpful, or unsatisfying. This indicates your level of relationship satisfaction, relationship strain, social inclusion, or exclusion.

How's the quality of your social connections? How many close friends do you have, ones with whom you share the most intimate details of your life? Are most of your relationships positive, helpful, and satisfying? If not, why not?

_____

_____

Which quality relationships would you like to deepen further? How could you set that in motion?

_____

_____

Do you have dysfunctional relationships that you'd like to improve? Which ones can you address and work on improving? How would you approach each person?

_____

_____

LONELY PEOPLE DIE EARLY

In a meta-analysis of studies on loneliness, researchers found that living with air pollution increases your odds of dying early by 5 percent; living with obesity by 20 percent; excessive drinking by 30 percent; and loneliness by a whopping 45 percent.

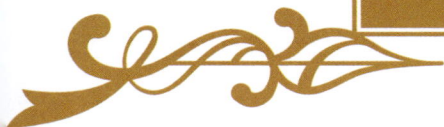

WHO'S IN YOUR CIRCLES?

According to British evolutionary psychologist Dr. Robin Dunbar, we have "circles of friendships." If you place yourself in the center of the circle, the inner circle are your *qualitative or intimate friendships*, with whom you share the deepest bonds of mutual affection and trust. These are romantic partners, family, and close friends, our strongest emotional bonds, who provide ongoing protection, support, and emotional sustenance. The middle circle would be your *functional friendships*, people who offer shared support and connection, primarily on a reciprocal basis. We don't rely on them, but know they would step up, if needed. The outer circle would be *structural friends*, members of a larger community, neighbors, colleagues, classmates, and acquaintances who help you feel part of a collective. Dr. Dunbar says that we allocate some 60 percent of our interpersonal time and energy to our inner circle, typically less than five people. While he warns that relationships with the inner circle or "core people" will wither without direct, face-to-face communication that allows all to be fully present and available to each other, it's also important that you foster other friendships. It's also crucial that you resolve conflicts and actively nurture relationships, particularly with your inner circle.

Who is in your inner, intimate circle? How are these relationships faring these days? Are you giving them your full attention and enough face-to-face time? With whom and in what ways do you need to strengthen these relationships?

_____

_____

_____

Who's in your middle, functional circle? Are you fostering those relationships, encouraging reciprocal mutuality? If not, why?

_____

_____

_____

Who's in your outer, structural circle? How can you expand and bolster those relationships?

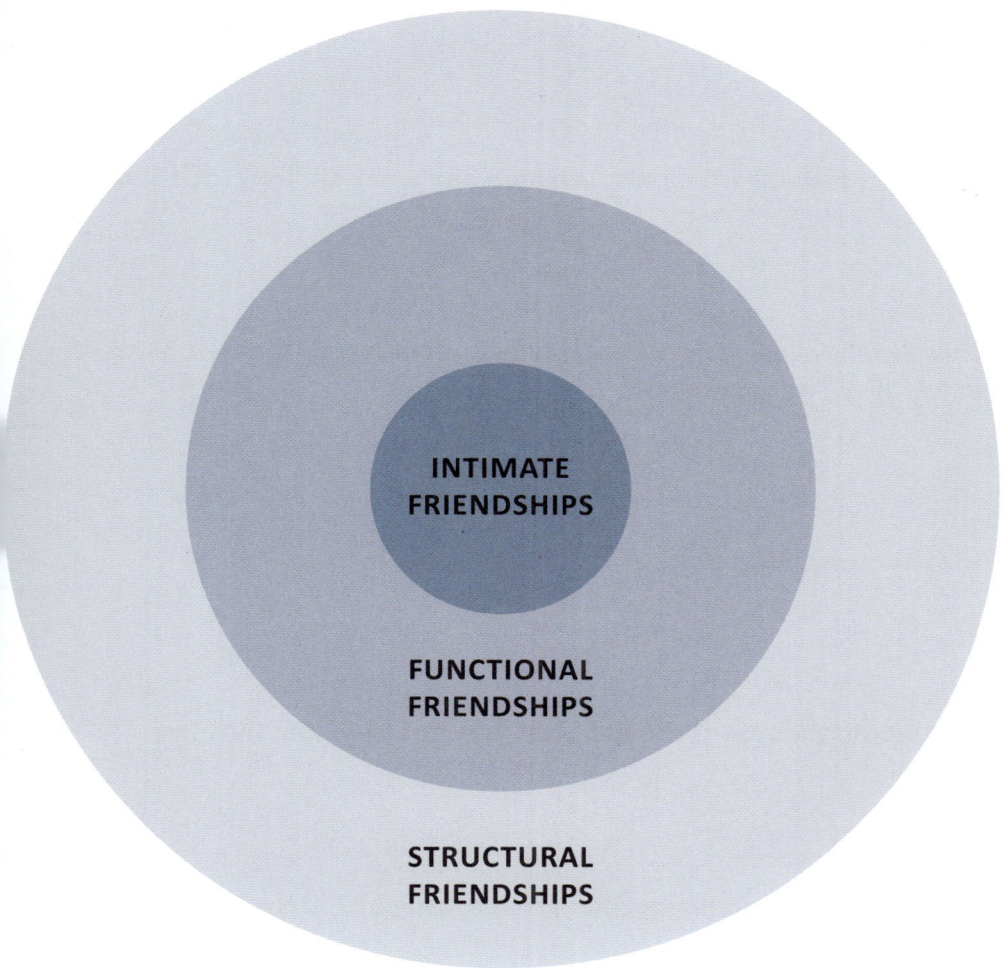

_____

_____

_____

_____

INTIMATE FRIENDSHIPS

FUNCTIONAL FRIENDSHIPS

STRUCTURAL FRIENDSHIPS

HOW WELL DO YOU KNOW YOUR FRIENDS?

To see how truly close you are to the friends around you, take this short quiz. Pick two or three close friends, write the names next to the first two or three numbers, and then answer each question for each friend.

Name three close friends:

1.   2.   3.

Questions to answer for each friend:
What is this person's current favorite food or place to dine out?

1.   2.   3.

Where did they take their last vacation and what did they love about it?

1.   2.   3.

What are they currently most enjoying (or hating) about their place of work/school/volunteerism?

1.   2.   3.

What are they most stressed out about at the moment?

1.   2.   3.

What would they say is the happiest event of their life, thus far?

1.   2.   3.

Who had the biggest impact on them growing up? In their early days at work/school?

1.   2.   3.

Are they happy in their work? What would be their ideal job or activity?

1.   2.   3.

What are the specific goals they're working towards now?

1.   2.   3.

If they suddenly got a large inheritance, how would they spend it?

1.   2.   3.

What do they consider their best traits? Worst habits?

1.   2.   3.

What do they feel most pride about doing or being?

1.   2.   3.

How did you do? If you found many questions difficult to answer, you may not be as close to these intimate friends as you think you are and need to work on deepening each relationship. Even if it's someone who's been around for a long time, ongoing intimacy through mutual sharing is something that needs to be nurtured and reinforced.

Were you surprised at how little you know about your best friends? What do you need to do to strengthen those relationships?

_____

_____

_____

_____

CONNECT WITH YOURSELF

When you feel 'less than' others and allow it to keep you from connecting with others, turn your attention inward. Instead of asking: Am I keeping up with whoever is in my social circles? Am I keeping up in a way that my mind says is comparable to others? Ask yourself: Am I being true to myself today? Have I been kind or a good friend to myself and others? Did I choose to act in ways consistent with what I value? Then give yourself credit for being true to yourself. Doing so will bolster a sense of self-efficacy, esteem, and comfort with who you are. Set aside at least five minutes a day (every day) to look inward, and meditate, pray, practice yoga, or read a couple of pages of a spiritual text.

What was revealed about your connection to yourself after reading and contemplating the depth of your relationships?

_____

_____

Write five good things about yourself that reflect how you feel about yourself.

1 _____

2 _____

3 _____

4 _____

5 _____

ARE YOU AN INTROVERT OR AN EXTROVERT?

According to founder of analytical psychology Carl Jung, extroverts typically feel energized by being surrounded by people, enjoy interacting with the outside world, and prefer sharing their thoughts and feelings with others, while introverts typically feel recharged by being alone, feel most secure and confident in their own space, and like opportunities to contemplate quietly in a serene place. So, which are you? Answer yes or no to the following questions:

1. Do you enjoy spending time alone, focused on your own thoughts?
2. Does being alone help you recharge?
3. Do you prefer activities or hobbies that take place in a small, quiet setting?
4. Does being at a crowded party make you uncomfortable?
5. Do you avoid meeting new people and feel drained after socializing?
6. Do you spend more time listening than talking?
7. Do you feel uncomfortable when the spotlight is on you?
8. Do you initiate conversations, or wait for someone to talk to you?
9. Do you enjoy socializing with various kinds of people, most of whom you don't know?
10. Does being around other people, exploring new places, or experiencing lively environments make you feel energized?
11. Are you broad-minded, easy to approach, and comfortable in most social situations?
12. Do you find it easy to talk to almost anyone, about almost anything?
13. Are you always game for a social outing?
14. Do you often initiate conversations with others?
15. Do you prefer to talk about yourself rather than listen to someone else ramble on?
16. Do you enjoy being the center of attention?

If you answered yes to questions 1-8, you are more introverted; and if you answered yes to questions 8-16, you are more extroverted, but being extroverted does not mean that you aren't lonely.

How do you feel about being an introvert or an extrovert? What qualities of either concern you? Do you want to expand how you think about yourself, how you choose to interact with others?

_____

_____

_____

How does this tendency reflect the closeness and frequency of any social engagement?

_____

_____

_____

Do you want to move in one direction or the other? What would it take to do so?

_____

_____

_____

EVEN EXTROVERTS GET LONELY

Extroverts are often surrounded by others and may have many friends, but they may not form deep attachments. Also, because they love being around other people, tend to keep the spotlight on themselves, and derive both affirmation and energy from socializing, they may find being alone stressful and may feel lonelier than introverts when alone. And, contrary to what many may assume, because they are comfortable being alone with only their own thoughts, an introvert may rarely feel lonely.

Do you tend to have introverts or extroverts as friends? If so, how does their method of attachment affect the level of intimacy between you? What would you like to change?

_____

_____

If you're an extrovert, do you often feel lonely? Is it because you keep relationships at a surface level? What could you do to change this?

_____

_____

INTROVERTS ARE SOCIAL BEINGS

Perhaps surprisingly, introverts may ultimately be the more social beings, because:

- They prefer having a smaller, select group of friends with whom they can share and discuss what's important to them, as well as their vulnerabilities.
- They socialize with fewer people, but, once acquainted, introverts often form longer-lasting, more intimate relationships.
- They pay attention when others talk, avoid conflict, and think about their words and actions, which shows consideration for others.
- They take time to build friendships, invest more energy in forming attachments, and, once they establish mutual trust, offer a true, reciprocal friendship.

If you're an introvert, how does what you read make you feel? If you're an extrovert, which qualities might you want to bolster?

_____

_____

_____

BEING AMBIVERT IS BEST

While there's nothing wrong with being an introvert or an extrovert. Ideally you want to be an ambivert, someone who has both introverted and extroverted attributes. Ambiverts:

- Feel energized when socializing but also enjoy solitude
- Tend to be highly adaptable, flexible, and capable of striking a balanced social life
- Both listen and speak well, making them compatible with introverts, extroverts, and other personality types
- Are typically flexible in their thinking, tend to be good natured, and are both empathetic and supportive.

What are some ways you could channel your natural or habitual tendencies into being an ambivert?

_____

_____

What are some of the challenges you'll need to overcome in order to be more of an ambivert? How will you address them?

_____

_____

"If you're lonely
when you're alone,
you're in bad company."

— JEAN-PAUL SARTRE

EMBRACE HUGS

Everyone benefits physically, mentally, emotionally, and spiritually from closeness and intimacy. Your brain responds to close interaction by releasing oxytocin, the 'feel-good' hormone, which further increases social bonds. If you don't have an intimate partner in your life, even a six-second hug from someone can spur oxytocin release. The more fully (or tightly) you embrace, the better.

QUALITY TRUMPS QUANTITY

Research shows that you reap the psychological well-being and physical health benefits of social connection not from the number of friends you have, but from the depth of your internal and subjective sense of connection toward others. It's the quality of your connections, not the number.

HOW LONELY ARE YOU?

Even the loneliest people don't tend to view their condition as problematic. You could feel lonely often and still not recognize it as something you need to address. Let's take a quiz to see if you're lonelier than you think.

Take the Loneliness Quiz

Answer the following yes or no questions. Do not include your spouse, or significant other, as a friend.

Do you talk to someone daily?   Y   N

Are you often by yourself and bored?   Y   N

Does being alone make you anxious?   Y   N

Do you often feel out of sorts?   Y   N

Do you have friends with similar interests?   Y   N

Do you regularly make time to enjoy activities with friends?   Y   N

Do you have three, or more, close personal friendships in which you are truly authentic?   Y   N

Do you have long conversations with friends on a regular basis?   Y   N

Do you talk with friends in depth about your personal issues?   Y   N

Are you close to your siblings or other family members?   Y   N

Do you make time to see family often?   Y   N

Do you offer them your full attention when present?   Y   N

Do you have close friends at work?   Y   N

Do you invite coworkers to socialize outside of work?   Y   N

Do you trust anyone at work with your secrets?   Y   N

Do you make new friends easily?   Y   N

Do you tend to avoid parties and other social events?   Y   N

Are you able to be vulnerable in relationships?   Y   N

Are you experiencing conflict in important relationships?   Y   N

Do you feel like your friends appreciate you?   Y   N

Do you have someone you feel truly understands you?   Y   N

If you are in an emotional crisis, do you have friends you can call?   Y   N

Do you have a faith-based community?   Y   N

Do you spend too much time isolated or alone?   Y   N

Would you rather be alone than with others?   Y   N

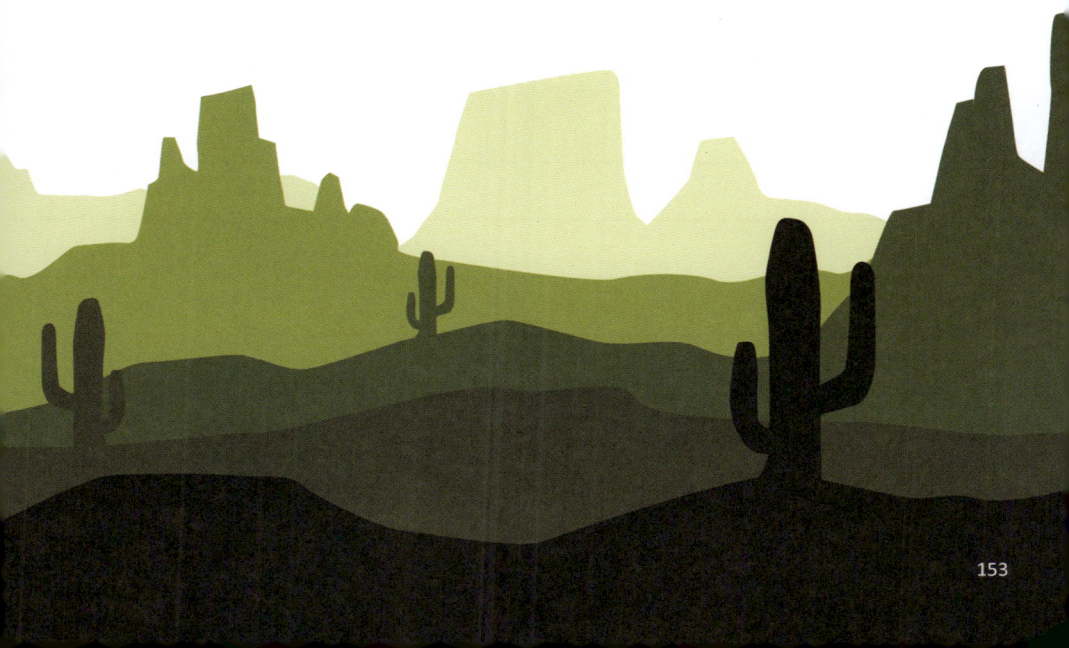

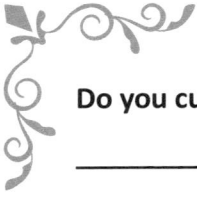

Do you currently have a loneliness problem**? Why or why not?**

_____

_____

_____

_____

_____

Which of the questions best identified **your problem areas?**

_____

_____

_____

_____

_____

Which of those are you most concerned **about?**

_____

_____

_____

_____

_____

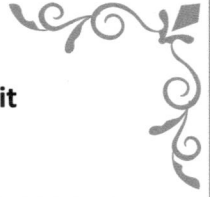

When you're feeling lonely, how do you comfort yourself? Is it effective?

_____

_____

_____

_____

_____

_____

_____

If you're not reaching out to others to form deeper connections, why not?

_____

_____

_____

_____

_____

_____

_____

_____

START *NOW* TO WIDEN AND STRENGTHEN YOUR SOCIAL NETWORK

Social engagement offers a multifaceted protective effect across all domains of healthy aging. It significantly enhances mental health by reducing stress, anxiety, and depression, fostering a sense of belonging, and stimulating positive emotions. It also sharpens cognitive function by constantly challenging and engaging the brain, strengthening neural pathways, and improving working memory, processing speed, and verbal fluency. Studies indicate that socially active seniors are less likely to develop dementia and other cognitive decline-related conditions and have as much as a greater chance of living longer than those who are not socially active.

Don't wait to make friends down the road. Get started *now* on creating and strengthening your social network. If you need ideas for making that happen, here are a few:

- **Make the effort to reach out.** Phones and social media have given us a false sense of social discourse. Spending time face-to-face (hug-to-hug) strengthens relationships. Make time in your busy schedule to make and deepen friendships and alliances.

- **Seek opportunities to connect.** Attend events, church, or community activities. Look for classes or groups with people who have interests similar to yours.

- **Find a cause or two and volunteer.** Volunteering not only improves your physical and mental health; it provides a sense of purpose. It's also a great way to build new relationships.

- **Extend and accept invitations.** An invitation to meet for coffee or go for a walk around the neighborhood may brighten someone else's day as much as it does yours.

- **Be fully present.** Relationships take time and effort. Whether connecting with a friend you've known for a long time or someone you just met, be fully present in the moment, and offer your full attention to the person and situation.

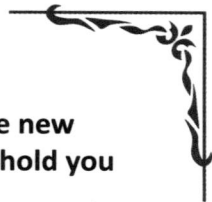

If you've been slow to reach out to friends or trying to make new friends, why? Are there feelings of insecurity or doubt that hold you back? Do these reasons still have a reason to exist?

_____

_____

Think back to the last time you tried to make a new friend and write about that experience. If it went well, note why you think it worked and give yourself kudos; if it didn't go well, explore why.

_____

_____

What did you do that specifically strengthened that burgeoning relationship?

_____

_____

What are interests that you'd like to spend more time exploring? Is there a new hobby you've always wanted to explore, such as gardening, bird-watching, quilting, golf, or travel photography? Identify a few interests below and then look for opportunities in your area to join groups doing the things you'd like to explore.

_____

_____

KEY TAKEAWAYS FOR *EXPAND YOUR WORLD: CULTIVATE RELATIONSHIPS*

- Strong social relationships are vital to healthy aging, offering emotional and practical support that boosts happiness, reduces stress, and lowers risks of depression, cognitive decline, and chronic illness. According to Mayo Clinic experts, the quality and depth of your interpersonal connections—more than genetics or physical health—play the greatest role in aging well.

- Our friendships are organized in circles: a small inner circle of close, intimate relationships including family and romantic partners, a middle circle of functional friendships offering reciprocal support, and a larger outer circle of acquaintances providing a sense of community. We typically spend about 60 percent of our social engagement nurturing the inner circle, which usually includes fewer than five people, and these core bonds require face-to-face interaction, conflict resolution, and ongoing care to remain strong.

- Social engagement supports healthy aging by reducing mental health issues, enhancing cognitive function, and increasing longevity, with socially active seniors showing lower risks of dementia and cognitive decline. To build and maintain meaningful connections, prioritize face-to-face interactions, seek community activities, volunteer, accept and extend invitations, and be fully present in your relationships.

"Old friends pass away, new friends appear…
The important thing is to make it meaningful:
a meaningful friend—or a meaningful day."

— HIS HOLINESS, THE DALAI LAMA

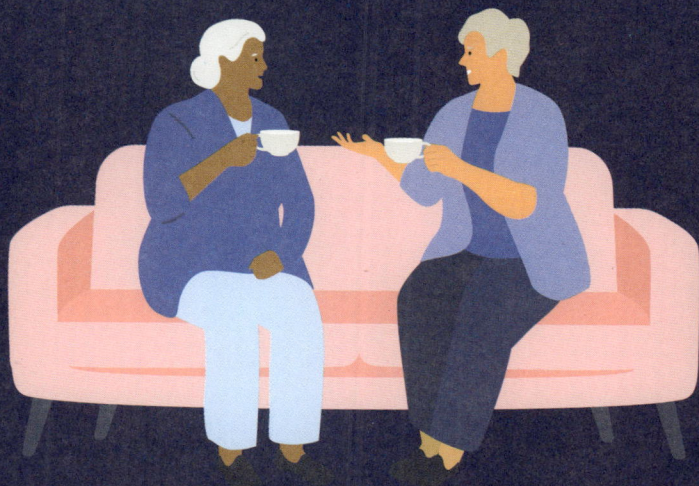

"I want to be the representation for women that your sexy never dies 'til you're in the box.' I decided that I wasn't going to allow the world, men, or this [film] industry to dictate how I live my life and how I age. I'm going to turn 50 just like I turned 30, except you know, my knees are a little different. I'm not going to buy into my career is over, or life for me is over, or sexy is over, or I shouldn't wear this. I'm going to do what I feel."

— Taraji P. Henson

Create a Vision
FOR YOUR FUTURE

Create a Vision for Your Future

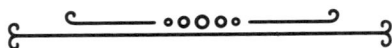

During early adulthood and well into middle age, most of us are focused on our careers, or at least making as much money as possible (and saving for retirement, hopefully). We can get so focused that we develop "success addiction," meaning we are too focused on work, to the detriment of quality of life and expansion. As we age, typically, inner fulfillment becomes more important. We may (and should!) assess where we are, what we've been doing, what's good or what's not working, and how we'd like to be living our lives as we age.

According to David Cravit and Larry Wolf, authors of *The Seven Essentials of Super Aging*, how you choose to age truly matters. They delineated two types of aging: default aging and what they call "superaging." Default aging is adhering to past experiences without recognizing that times have changed that the process of aging has changed. Like the ancestors who preceded them, those who cling to default aging enter their elder years *expecting* to experience decline. They accept old ways of thinking that predicted their aging process would involve:

- Retirement from the professional and gradually the social world
- A drastic curtailment in spending
- The end of romance and sex
- A steady physical and mental decline
- Little to no meaningful additions to their accomplishments.

Superagers, on the other hand, enter their elder years fully expecting to enjoy and foster continued health, activity, and growth well into old age. Whereas default agers see their elder years as full of the kind of long, slow decline that leads to death, superagers see their elder years as *full of opportunity* to live a healthy, active, exciting life. Superagers stay focused on life. They know they'll die . . . *someday* . . . but they intend to live life as fully as possible until a more sudden death calls.

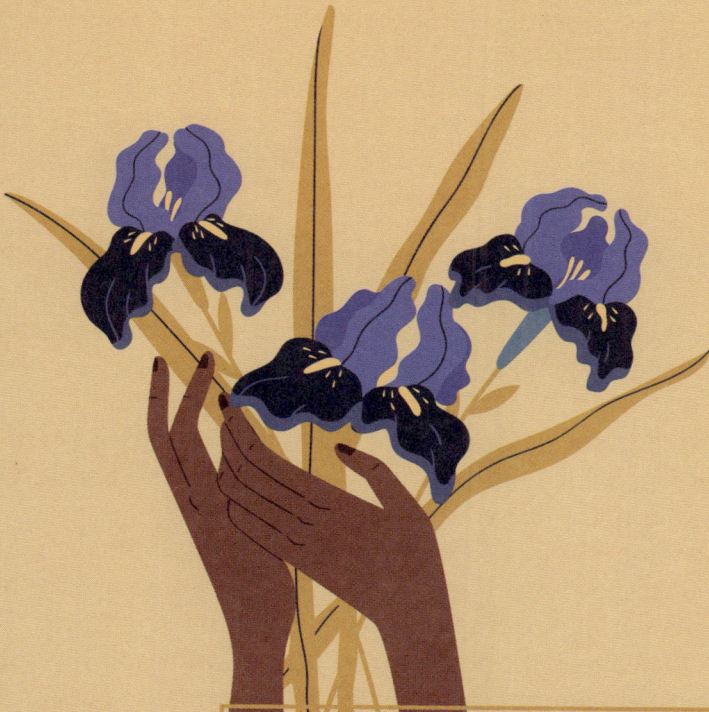

BUILD THAT NEST EGG

Have you heard of the 4 percent rule? To cover thirty years of retirement, financial consultants say you should ideally only take a 4 percent distribution each year from your IRA or pension. Unfortunately, they base this percentage on the premise that you'll have at least $1 million in retirement funds upon retirement. If you do have a million, that means $40,000 a year in income; as a point of reference, most Baby Boomers have around $250,000 upon retirement, 4 percent of which is approximately $8,000 a year, which is pretty hard to live on. It's necessary and wise to beef up your retirement savings now.

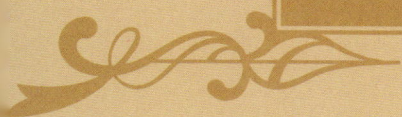

Cravit and Wolf identified what they call seven critical pillars that, collectively, help us transition from a narrow, default aging mindset to a wider, more exciting mindset towards superaging. Here's seven pillars they say you need to master to become a superager. Note that each of the following seven steps work synergistically, by reinforcing each other:

1. Attitude. Maintain an optimistic mindset, be enthusiastic about your future.
2. Awareness. Become an active seeker and consumer of information relevant to healthy aging, then use that knowledge to bolster your health.
3. Activity. Be fully aware of the need to keep your body and brain healthy, keep an open, eager attitude towards activities that foster physical, emotional, and mental health.
4. Accomplishment. Plan ahead to transition from a full-time job into a suitable course of activity that provides a sense of accomplishment, and often money. Set goals and work towards achieving them.
5. Autonomy. Plan ahead for financial and physical autonomy. Practice good money management and seek resources to meet your current and future needs.
6. Attachment. Stay emotionally attached to family and friends while also reaching out to new people and situations. Initiate and maintain ongoing social interaction
7. Avoidance. Avoid or challenge anything that causes self-defeating perceptions or actions. Flip negatives to positives.

What's your honest assessment **of how you are doing on each? Where are your strengths? Where do you need to improve? Be specific, give yourself credit for your strengths, and then list ways you can immediately bolster areas where you need to improve.**

_____

_____

_____

_____

_____

_____

_____

_____

_____

_____

_____

_____

"I think acting your age means
that you've stopped being curious about
not just your present, but your future, too,
and you're allowing other people to dictate
your life experience for you. So, let's just stop
trying to turn back the clock, shall we?"

— ALAN CUMMING

PLAN AHEAD FOR YOUR THIRD ACT

Unless they suffer catastrophic health, people who reach the age of sixty-five can reasonably expect to live, on average, at least two more decades. As most people still retire right around the age of sixty-five, they have twenty *to thirty* more years in which to do something beyond work, something completely new and exciting, something that challenges and stimulates them, something, perhaps, that they've always wanted to do but never had the time.

Now that you've let that settle, isn't it odd that people typically go into retirement with only a slight plan of what they'll do or how they'll live their life? They look forward to not having to work a demanding, structured job every day, but they haven't thought through what they will do with their time, what they might *need to do*, or *truly want* to do with their time. They just presume they'll feel free and happy. The initial stages of retirement may validate those expectations, but those who haven't created a vision or concrete plan for the next twenty years of their lives, may soon feel disenchanted, disappointed, bored, isolated, rudderless, and lost.

To successfully navigate retirement, you need meaning and purpose, to find things to do that bolster your sense of self, empowerment, and value. Without a plan for making your third act vital, active, and meaningful, you are more likely to fall into despair, loneliness, and depression.

In order to best serve its aging clients, investment firm JP Morgan Chase & Co. now tells its managers to create financial plans for healthy, nonsmoking clients with the premise that they will live to one hundred. They are instructed to presume that those aging now will fully optimize their later stages of life.

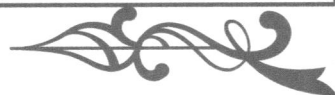

Now that you've had time to work through this book, what have you identified in terms of your values and desires that will determine how you live and what you do post-retirement and well into your eighties?

Do you plan to simply cut back on hours or find a new job? If you want to create a new career post-retirement, what are three alternatives to explore?

1 _____

2 _____

3 _____

If you want to get additional education, what fields hold the most appeal?

_____

_____

If you want to work part-time outside your current field, how many hours and in what field?

_____

_____

If you want to volunteer, what and where do you think you'll find rewarding opportunities?

_____

_____

If you want to travel, how will you support that lifestyle? What would be your ideal destination?

_____

_____

REIMAGINE YOUR FUTURE

According to Daniel H. Pink, author of *From Strength to Strength,* letting go of attachment to achievement and turning towards wisdom, relationships with others, and spiritual growth require an aging person to "reimagine the rest of his or her life."

In other words, you need to form a new identity and the attitude necessary to fully embrace and inhabit it. This can only happen if you:

- Find purpose and meaning outside of work
- Consciously contemplate your third act and explore options
- Build enthusiasm for new life choices
- Open yourself to new ideas
- Create a viable and dynamic plan for aging gracefully
- Prepare for change
- Actively manage your future.

CONTEMPLATING CHANGE

Reimagining your life simply means sitting down long enough to contemplate how you want your later years to manifest. Giving deep thought to how you will approach and live your later years will boost positive feelings and give you something to look forward to.

1. Determine what needs to change or how you wish things to change. Perhaps it's continuing to work well into your seventies, or cutting back on work rather than retiring? Or perhaps it's pursuing a whole new career or venture. Perhaps it's creating a nonprofit or volunteering at your local hospital.
2. Determine the values that are most important to you, especially those relevant to feeling useful and fulfilled in this upcoming, new phase of life. Refer to the values list on page 127 and decide which values will most nourish your soul as you age?
3. Create concrete goals based on those values. Create a mental map of what is needed to live the imagined life, and then create goals designed to achieve whatever is needed. Make the goals pertinent to your values so they will have meaning and purpose.

4. Research possibilities. Make a list of options, then explore each in depth. Determine which ones are more suited to your desires and are achievable. Possibly create a list of steps you'll need to take to reach those goals (learning a new skill or more schooling, as examples).

5. Consider hiring a life coach. When making long-range plans, it may be helpful to have an objective person who can help you explore and then narrow down your options.

Considering what we've discussed in terms of reimagining your future, what do you need to change to live a happier, healthier, more fulfilling life, both now and in the distant future?

_____

_____

_____

_____

_____

_____

_____

_____

_____

_____

_____

_____

_____

_____

_____

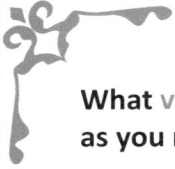

What values [see page 127] are most important to you, particularly as you mature? What will ultimately make your life feel meaningful?

_____

_____

What are three goals you are currently pursuing?

1 _____

2 _____

3 _____

Which of the three is most important to you? Why?

_____

_____

_____

Which of the goals carries the most heat? Gets you excited?

_____

_____

_____

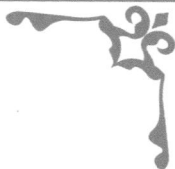

Which feels like it would be most fulfilling?

_____

_____

_____

What are five possibilities you will commit to exploring as options for your third act?

1 _____

2 _____

3 _____

4 _____

5 _____

How will you begin to explore your chosen options? List specific steps you will commit to taking.

_____

_____

_____

ENVISION YOUR FUTURE SELF

Imagine for a moment that you are living a 'well-lived' life at age eighty. What would that life look like? What would you have done in your sixties and seventies that bolstered this new life? Where would you be? What would you be doing? Who would be around you? How would your body and soul be feeling? Would you feel fulfilled, energetic, happy? Write a few paragraphs that describe your imagined life. Write it the way you'd most want it to look and feel.

WRITE TO YOUR FUTURE SELF

Write a letter to the self you want to be twenty or thirty years down the road. Think about how choices you've made along the way have affected who you've become. Take pride in your growth process and then inform the *future you* how you expect to live your life, what you want to be doing at that age, how you are setting the stage now and will reap the benefits later. Reaffirm how you will positively view your aging self and be sure to promise *future you* that will hold yourself in high esteem throughout the aging process.

KEY TAKEAWAYS FOR *CREATE A VISION FOR YOUR FUTURE*

- During middle age, many become overly focused on career success, often neglecting inner fulfillment, which means reassessing priorities becomes crucial. 'Default aging' involves expecting decline and withdrawal, while 'superaging' embraces continued health, activity, and growth, viewing later years as a time of opportunity and full living.

- The seven interconnected pillars of superaging are: maintaining a positive attitude, actively seeking knowledge about healthy aging, engaging in physical and mental activities, pursuing meaningful accomplishments, ensuring financial and physical autonomy, nurturing social connections, and avoiding self-defeating behaviors. Together, these pillars support a broader, more empowered approach to aging that fosters health, purpose, and connection.

- Aging requires reimagining your life by letting go of achievement-focused identity and embracing purpose, relationships, and growth through conscious planning and openness to change. This involves deeply contemplating desired changes, identifying core values, setting meaningful goals, exploring options, and potentially seeking guidance via a life coach to actively manage your future.

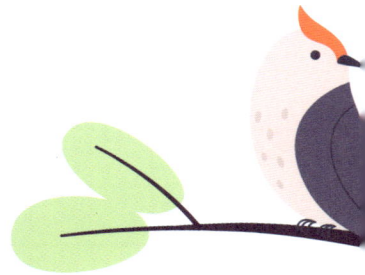

"My position has always been that the way people age and the signs that we show of aging is nature's way of tattooing. It's natural scarification, and the life you lead gives you the symbols and the emblems of your life, the road map you followed."

— Frances McDormand

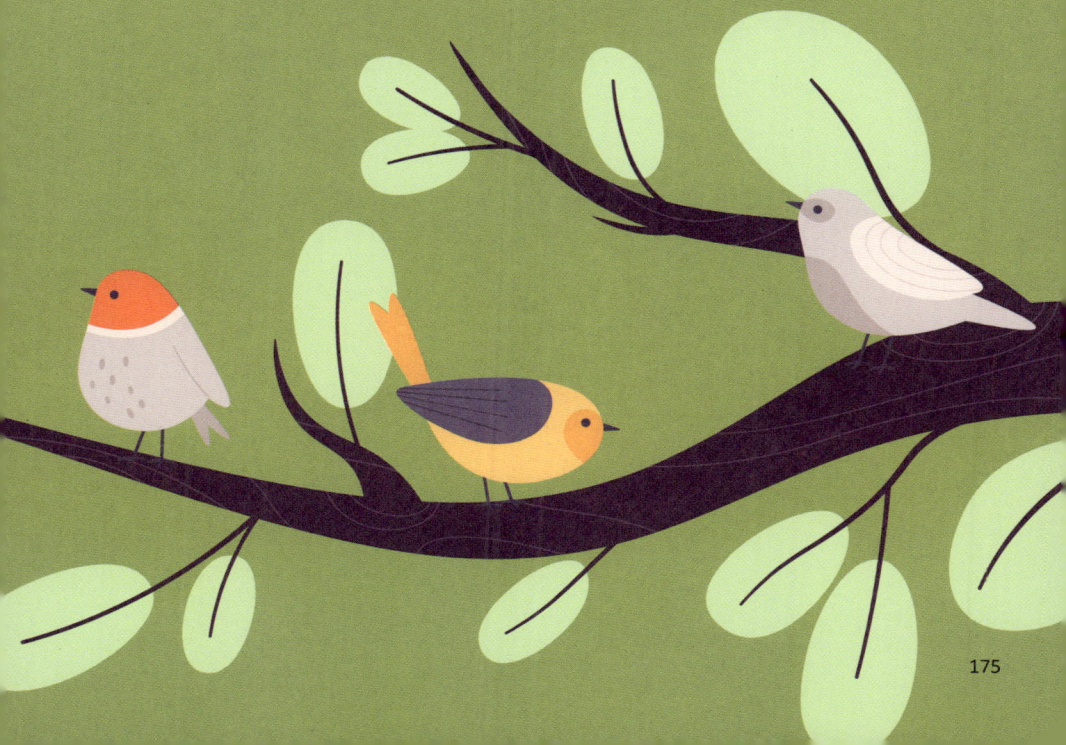

"I'm probably not a great person to ask about age because I never lie about my age, I love my age. Even when I was younger, I'd look in the face of Helen Mirren and Jane Fonda and Cicely Tyson, and all I'd see was beauty. But yes, the industry does put a lot of pressure on you. There's a feeling like you're no longer valuable when you get older. I don't feel that our society has embraced what comes with aging. They think that you just get old, we don't value wisdom, and we don't value experience. Our business is very much image-conscious, then you have societal pressure on people, then you have a perfect storm of there being a lot of age discrimination. But this is where I think midlife crisis comes into play. It's about liberating yourself from all of that."

— VIOLA DAVIS

PRIORITIZE
Joy

Prioritize Joy

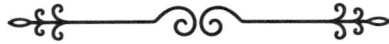

Just as we naturally and later purposefully learn to lift and stretch our body to maintain flexibility, we can learn to lift and expand our spirits to keep it youthful. A youthful spirit is lighthearted, full of forgiveness, playfulness, curiosity, awe, and wonder. Being wise, patient, and kind, expressing love and forgiveness to others, fostering happiness and joy, and embracing change all cultivate a youthful spirit.

So, how do you develop and maintain a youthful spirit? Here are some ideas.

- **Learn to love change:** Rather than fear or resist change, embrace every opportunity for growth.
- **Practice lifelong learning:** Keep your mind engaged by expanding your knowledge and learning new skills.
- **Try new things:** Step outside your comfort zone, experiment with activities and hobbies.
- **Focus on the positive aspects of life.** Maintain an optimistic outlook.
- **Get lots of exercise:** Boost your mood and energy levels via exercise.
- **Nourish body and brain:** Eat a balanced diet rich in fruits, vegetables, and whole grains.
- **Make time for joy:** Make time for laughter and activities that bring you genuine happiness.
- **Practice mindfulness:** Practice being fully present in the moment to appreciate life as it unfolds.
- **Strengthen social connections:** Maintain close personal relationships with friends and family
- **Cultivate positive qualities:** Practice kindness, compassion, patience, and empathy.

Which of the qualities mentioned do you most need to cultivate or expand? How will you foster your youthful spirit going forward?

_____

_____

_____

_____

_____

_____

_____

_____

_____

_____

_____

_____

_____

_____

CONSIDER YOURSELF BORN AGAIN

In Japan, old age is seen as a spring or rebirth after a busy period of working and raising children. The elderly are also revered and often live with family. One study found older adults in Japan showed higher scores on personal growth compared with midlife adults, whereas the opposite age pattern was found in the United States.

LEARN TO PLAY

Playfulness is one way individuals (re)frame situations in such a way that they experience events as intellectually stimulating and/or entertaining and/or personally interesting. Playfulness becomes a resource for coping with challenges and life events common in later life, such as transitioning from work to retirement, health issues, and loss. Playfulness in adults between the ages of fifty and ninety-eight years has been found to be similar to the playfulness children experience and that being playful builds character strengths, contributes positively to life satisfaction, bolsters a sense of well-being, and helps one flourish.

What do you currently do to have fun? What do you enjoy most?

_____

_____

_____

_____

_____

_____

With whom among your circle of family and friends do you most enjoy playfulness? How does it manifest?

_____

_____

_____

_____

_____

_____

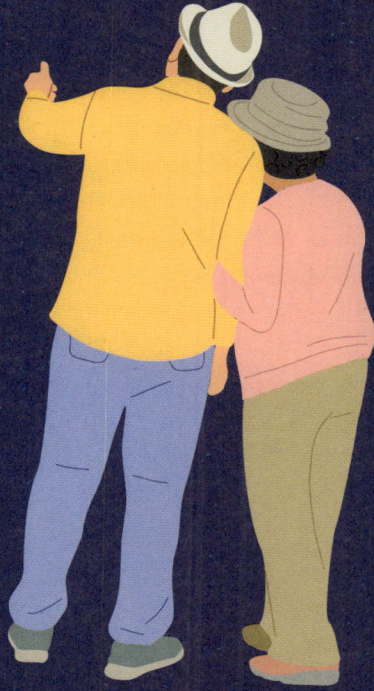

"As you get older; you've probably noticed that you tend to forget things. You'll be talking with somebody at a party, and you'll know that you know this person, but no matter how hard you try, you can't remember his or her name. This can be very embarrassing, especially if he or she turns out to be your spouse."

— DAVE BARRY

"We don't stop playing because we get old;
we grow old because we stop playing."

— GEORGE BARNARD SHAW

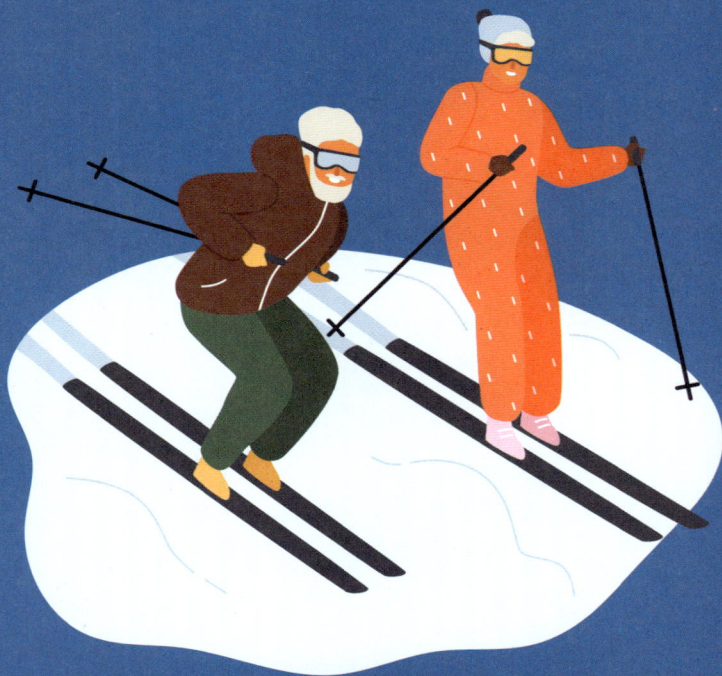

EXPLORE NEW HOBBIES

Studies have found that older people who have hobbies experience lower rates of depression. A study conducted during the pandemic found that people who started gardening, crafting, or woodworking for just 30 minutes a day reported greater life satisfaction than those who spend most of their time in front of TV screens or on their phones.

Jasmine Cho, author of *Get a Hobby*, defines a hobby as any activity that "grounds you in joy, can help you cope with sorrow, and can help you escape from life's burdens." She listed her hobbies as journaling, doodling, boxing, Legos, and puzzles, all of which help her achieve a state of flow that equates to getting lost, or even hyper-focused, which is the reward.

Do you have any hobbies now? What are they, what do you love about them?

_____

_____

_____

_____

_____

_____

What new hobbies could you explore?

_____

_____

_____

_____

_____

_____

_____

SEEK PLEASURE

When you're experiencing pleasure, your brain releases oxytocin and endorphins (known as the happy chemicals). Learning what makes you happy will serve you well now and as you age. Make pleasure seeking a habit.

Think of activities that make you happy, such as:

Listening to music: Music increases oxytocin levels in your brain, increases stamina, and enhances mood.

Going for a hike: Many studies have found that feeling connected to nature is positively correlated with feeling happy and having a sense of well-being.

Taking a yoga class: Yoga boosts endorphins in your brain and thereby helps reduce depression, anxiety, and stress, while concurrently improving sleep and enhancing overall quality of life.

Going out to dinner: Having a stimulating conversation while enjoying delicious food boosts oxytocin levels, and you get to enjoy all those sensory goodies, too.

Now think of five more activities that make you happy:

1 _____

2 _____

3 _____

4 _____

5 _____

Write a commitment to yourself about what you will do to seek pleasure and make yourself happier.

_____

_____

_____

_____

_____

_____

_____

_____

_____

_____

"Nothing is inherently and invincibly young except spirit. And spirit can enter a human being perhaps better in the quiet of old age and dwell there more undisturbed than in the turmoil of adventure."

— GEORGE SANTAYANA

FIND JOY EVERYWHERE

A recent study published in the *Journal of Neuroscience* found that older people feel less stress and regret, dwell less on negative information and are better able to regulate their emotions. Yes, older people face many challenges: health issues, cognitive decline, the loss of spouses and independence and yet this study (and others) reveal that life satisfaction and emotional stability begin to *increase* around the age of fifty-five. Though life satisfaction does begin to stabilize or even decline after age seventy, people over ninety years of age still report higher psychological wellbeing than their middle-aged counterparts! [*Age-Related Enhancements in Positive Emotionality across The Life Span: Structural Equation Modeling of Brain and Behavior:* Jason Stretton, Susanne Schweizer and Tim Dalgleish *Journal of Neuroscience* 20 April 2022]

What brings you joy now? List five things that excite joy in your life.

1 _____

2 _____

3 _____

4 _____

5 _____

> "Our goal shouldn't be to cling to youth as we get older, but to keep our joy alive by tending our inner child throughout our days, while also nurturing our connection to the changing world. In doing so, we balance wisdom with wonder, confidence with curiosity, and depth with delight."
>
> — INGRID FETELL LEE, JOYFUL: *THE SURPRISING POWER OF ORDINARY THINGS TO CREATE EXTRAORDINARY HAPPINESS*

Think of five things (or activities) that leave you awestruck.

1 _____

2 _____

3 _____

4 _____

5 _____

How can you incorporate more joy into your life?

_____

_____

If you need inspiration, check out *The School of Joy* website *aestheticsofjoy.com*.

GO ON AN "AWE WALK"

In a 2020 study of older adults published on the American Psychological Association website, researchers found that taking an "awe walk," a walk specifically focused on attending to vast or inspiring things in the environment, increased joy and prosocial emotions (feelings like generosity and kindness) more than simply taking a stroll in nature. Interestingly, they also found that 'smile intensity,' a measure of how much the participants smiled, increased over the eight-week duration of the study. The walks were only fifteen minutes long, once a week, and were low impact. So, this is an easy way to create more joy in daily life as you age.

Study: Big smile, small self: Awe walks promote prosocial positive emotions in older adults

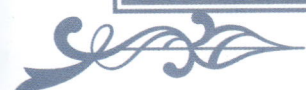

KEY TAKEAWAYS FOR *PRIORITIZE JOY*

- Playfulness can help reframe life's challenges in ways that feel stimulating, enjoyable, or meaningful. Research shows that older adults who embrace playfulness gain similar benefits to those seen in children—such as improved life satisfaction, character development, and a stronger sense of well-being.

- Engaging in hobbies also plays a crucial role in mental health during later life. Studies, including those conducted during the pandemic, found that activities like gardening, crafting, or woodworking—even for just thirty minutes a day—can significantly improve mood and life satisfaction compared to screen time.

- Pleasure-seeking habits like listening to music, spending time in nature, doing yoga, or socializing over dinner activate feel-good chemicals in the brain such as oxytocin and endorphins. Despite the many challenges of aging, studies show that emotional regulation, reduced stress, and increased psychological well-being often improve with age—especially after fifty-five—with even those over ninety reporting high levels of life satisfaction.

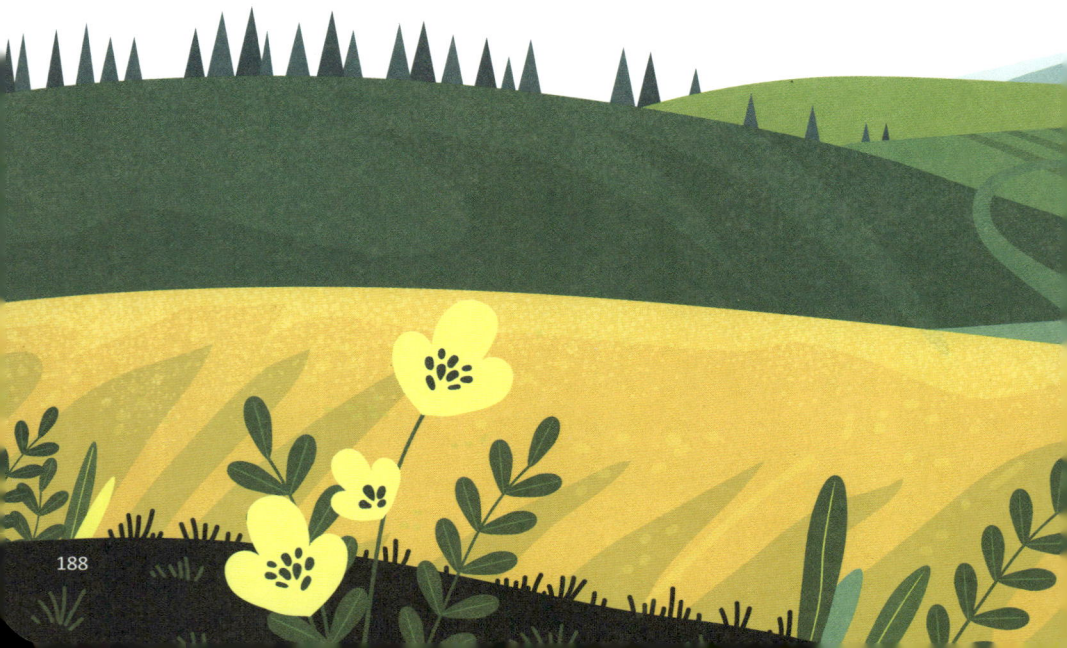

"Happiness is not a brilliant climax to years of grim struggle and anxiety. It is a long succession of little decisions simply to be happy in the moment."

— J. Donald Walters

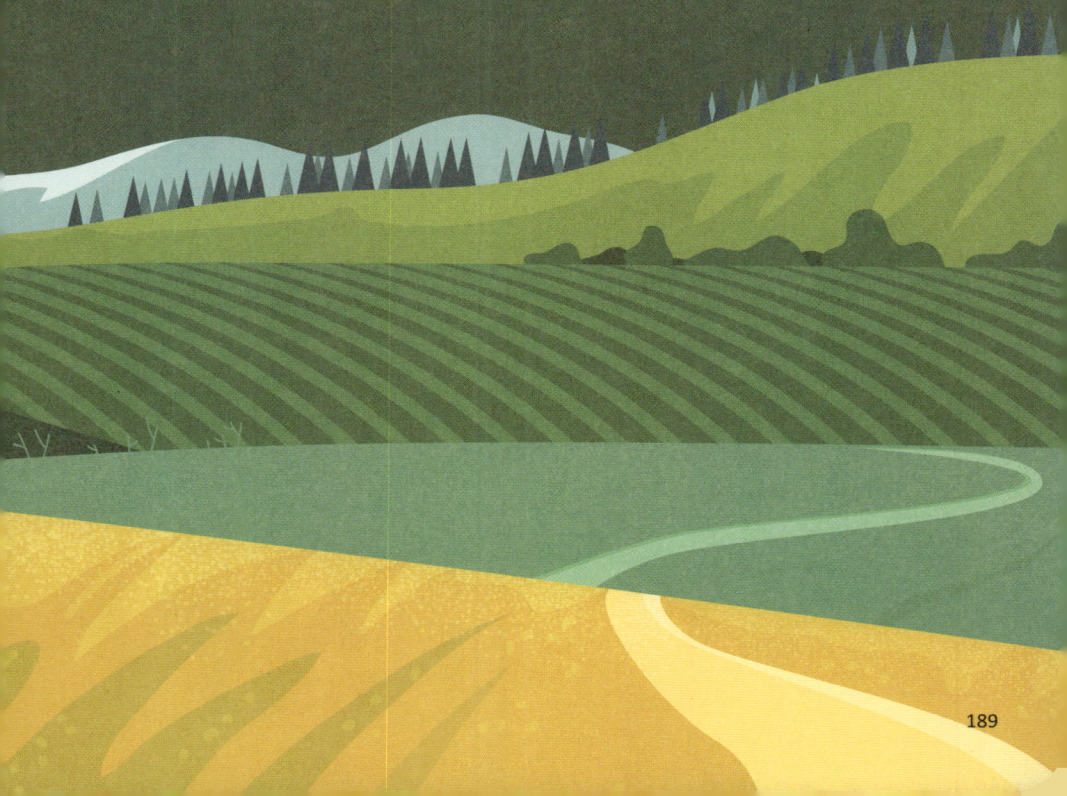

ARE YOU READY TO AGE GRACEFULLY?

We've reached the end of this journey, exploring where you are now to where you want to be when you've gracefully aged to a still-energetic, enthusiastic, and healthy ninety-five (or one hundred!).

Let's review the necessities of aging gracefully. To be your best, healthiest self as you age, you need to focus on three primary needs:

1. To *actively and habitually* maintain maximum overall health and physical functioning

2. To *actively and habitually* protect your brain and maintain cognitive functioning

3. To *actively and habitually* stay involved in social activities and productive pursuits.

We discussed and worked through a multitude of ways to achieve those three primary needs, and they include:

- Getting a new attitude about aging based on positivity
- Adjusting your habits to bolster efforts to maintain youthfulness
- Nourishing your body and brain through food choices and activity
- Finding purpose and meaning as motivation to stay engaged and active
- Cultivating and deepening relationships
- Creating a vision for your future that will re-energize you
- Prioritizing joy, playfulness, and pleasure.

Now that you've worked your way through all the prompts and exercises, how do you feel about your motivation to age gracefully? Are you fired up and ready to go?

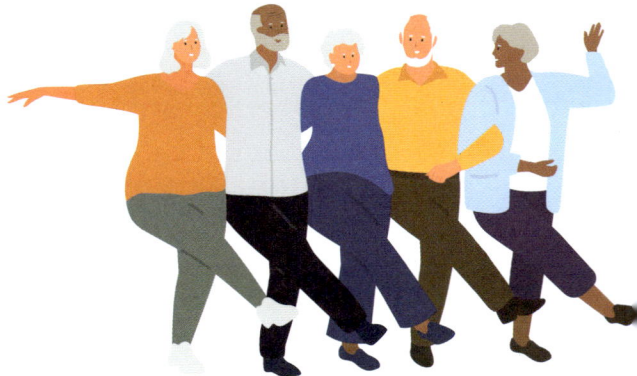

What are your biggest concerns or areas where you need the most improvement?

_____

_____

_____

_____

_____

What are five things you will immediately do to launch your *aging gracefully* journey?

1
_____

_____

2
_____

_____

3
_____

_____

4
_____

_____

5
_____

_____

Resources

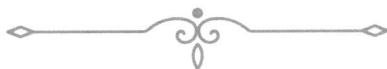

10 Keys to Happier Living: A Practical Handbook for Happiness, Vanessa King, Headline Publishing Group, 2016.

Breaking the Age Code: How Your Beliefs About Aging Determine How Long and Well You Live, Becca Levy, PhD.

Choose Your Life Purposes: A Step-by-Step Guide to Self-Awareness, Empowerment, and Success, Eric Maisel, PhD, Books That Save Lives, 2024.

Embrace Aging: Conquer Your Fears and Enjoy Added Years, Jeannette Guerrasio, MD, Rowan & Littlefield, 2022.

Growing Old: Notes on Aging with Something like Grace, Elizabeth Marshall Thomas, HarperOne, 2020.

Not Dead Yet: Rebooting Your Life after 50, Barbara Ballinger and Margaret Crane, Rowan & Littlefield, 2021.

Successful Aging: A Neuroscientist Explores the Power and Potential of Our Lives, Daniel Levitin.

The Ten Steps of Positive Ageing: A Handbook for Personal Change in Later Life, Guy Robertson.

Two Old Broads: Stuff You Need to Know That You Didn't Know You Needed to Know, Whoopi Goldberg and M.E. Hecht, MD, Harper Horizon, 2022.

You, Happier: The 7 Neuroscience Secrets of Feeling Good, Daniel G. Amen, MD, Tyndale Refresh, 2022.